The Rheumatoid Foot and Ankle

Guest Editor

LAWRENCE A. DIDOMENICO, DPM, FACFAS

CLINICS IN PODIATRIC MEDICINE AND SURGERY

www.podiatric.theclinics.com

Consulting Editor
THOMAS ZGONIS, DPM, FACFAS

April 2010 • Volume 27 • Number 2

SAUNDERS an imprint of ELSEVIER, Inc.

W.B. SAUNDERS COMPANY
A Division of Elsevier Inc.

1600 John F. Kennedy Boulevard • Suite 1800 • Philadelphia, Pennsylvania 19103-2899

http://www.theclinics.com

CLINICS IN PODIATRIC MEDICINE AND SURGERY Volume 27, Number 2
April 2010 ISSN 0891-8422, ISBN-13: 978-1-4377-1864-5

Editor: Patrick Manley

Clinics in Podiatric Medicine and Surgery (ISSN 0891-8422) is published quarterly by Elsevier Inc., 360 Park Avenue South, New York, NY 10010-1710. Months of issue are January, April, July, and October. Business and Editorial Offices: 1600 John F. Kennedy Blvd., Ste. 1800, Philadelphia, PA 19103-2899. Customer Service Office: 3251 Riverport Lane, Maryland Heights, MO 63043. Periodicals postage paid at New York, NY and additional mailing offices. Subscription prices are $252.00 per year for US individuals, $367.00 per year for US institutions, $130.00 per year for US students and residents, $303.00 per year for Canadian individuals, $454.00 for Canadian institutions, $359.00 for international individuals, $454.00 per year for international institutions and $184.00 per year for Canadian and foreign students/residents. To receive student/resident rate, orders must be accompanied by name of affiliated institution, date of term, and the *signature* of program/residency coordinator on institution letterhead. Orders will be billed at individual rate until proof of status is received. Foreign air speed delivery is included in all *Clinics* subscription prices. All prices are subject to change without notice. POSTMASTER: Send address changes to *Clinics in Podiatric Medicine and Surgery*, Elsevier Health Sciences Division, Subscription Customer Service, 3251 Riverport Lane, Maryland Heights, MO 63043. **Customer Service: 1-800-654-2452 (US). From outside of the US, call 314-447-8871. Fax: 314-447-8029. E-mail: JournalsCustomerService-usa@elsevier.com (for print support); JournalsOnlineSupport-usa@ elsevier.com (for online support).**

Reprints. For copies of 100 or more of articles in this publication, please contact the Commercial Reprints Department, Elsevier Inc., 360 Park Avenue South, New York, NY 10010-1710. Tel.: 212-633-3812; Fax: 212-462-1935; E-mail: reprints@elsevier.com.

Clinics in Podiatric Medicine and Surgery is covered in *MEDLINE/PubMed (Index Medicus)* and *EMBASE/Excerpta Medica.*

Printed and bound by CPI Group (UK) Ltd, Croydon, CR0 4YY

Transferred to Digital Print 2011

CLINICS IN PODIATRIC MEDICINE AND SURGERY

CONSULTING EDITOR
THOMAS ZGONIS, DPM, FACFAS

Contributors

CONSULTING EDITOR

THOMAS ZGONIS, DPM, FACFAS
Director, Podiatric Surgical Residency and Reconstructive Fellowship Programs;
Chief, Division of Podiatric Medicine and Surgery; Associate Professor, Department
of Orthopedic Surgery, The University of Texas Health Science Center at San Antonio,
San Antonio, Texas

GUEST EDITOR

LAWRENCE A. DIDOMENICO, DPM, FACFAS
Adjunct Professor, Ohio College of Podiatric Medicine; Director, Reconstructive Rearfoot
and Ankle Surgical Fellowship, Ankle and Foot Care Centers, Ohio College of Podiatric
Medicine; Section Chief of Podiatry, St Elizabeth's Medical Center, Youngstown, Ohio

AUTHORS

HEIKO ADAMS, DPM, FACFAS
Research Coordinator, Jewish Hospital and St Mary's Healthcare Podiatric Residency
Program, Louisville; Private Practice, Shelbyville, Kentucky; Diplomate of American Board
of Podiatric Surgery, Board Certified in Foot and Ankle Surgery

JOSEPH M. ANAIN Jr, DPM
Chairman, Department of Podiatry, Sisters Hospital; Director, Podiatric Medical
Education, Catholic Health System, Buffalo, New York

ANGELA R. BOJRAB, DPM
PGY-1, PM&S-24, Department of Podiatry, Catholic Health System, Buffalo, New York

LAURENCE Z. CAIN, DPM
Fellow, Reconstructive Rearfoot and Ankle Surgical Fellowship, Ankle and Foot Care
Centers/Ohio College of Podiatric Medicine, Youngstown, Ohio

MARC S. CO, DPM
Department of Orthopaedic Surgery, Kaiser Permanente Medical Group, Hayward/
Fremont California, Union City, California; PGY I, Kaiser Hayward PMS-36 Residency
Program, Hayward, California

LAWRENCE A. DIDOMENICO, DPM, FACFAS
Adjunct Professor, Ohio College of Podiatric Medicine; Director, Reconstructive Rearfoot
and Ankle Surgical Fellowship, Ankle and Foot Care Centers, Ohio College of Podiatric
Medicine; Chief, Section of Podiatry, St Elizabeth's Medical Center, Youngstown, Ohio

LAWRENCE HABER, MD
Associate Professor, Chief of Pediatric Orthopaedic Surgery, Department of Orthopaedic
Surgery, University of Mississippi Medical Center, Jackson, Mississippi

ALFONSO ANTHONY HARO III, DPM
Ankle and Foot Surgical and Podiatry Clinic, West End, North Carolina

ERNESTO S. HERNANDEZ, DPM
Department of Orthopaedic Surgery, Kaiser Permanente Medical Group, Hayward/Fremont California, Fremont; PGY III, Kaiser Hayward PMS-36 Residency Program, Hayward, California

ADAM HICKS, DPM
Fellow, Jewish Hospital and St Mary's Healthcare Podiatric Residency Program, Louisville, Kentucky

JOSHUA HUGHES, BA
Medical Student, School of Medicine, University of Mississippi Medical Center, Jackson, Mississippi

ALLEN MARK JACOBS, DPM, FACFAS, FAPWCA
St Louis, Missouri

ANASTASIOS D. KANELLOPOULOS, MD, DSC
First Department of Orthopaedics, Athens University Medical School, Athens, Greece

DEMETRIOS S. KORRES, MD
Third Department of Orthopaedics, Athens University Medical School, Kifisia, Athens, Greece

ANDREAS F. MAVROGENIS, MD
First Department of Orthopaedics, Athens University Medical School, Athens, Greece

EVANTHIA A. MITSIOKAPA, MD
Department of Physical Medicine and Rehabilitation, Thriasio Hospital, Elefsina, Greece

LACEY F. MOORE, MD
Pinehurst Radiology, Pinehurst, North Carolina

JASON D. NEUFELD, DPM
PGY II, Kaiser Hayward PMS-36 Residency Program, Hayward, California; Department of Orthopaedic Surgery, Kaiser Permanente Medical Group, Hayward/Fremont California, Union City, California

PANAYIOTIS J. PAPAGELOPOULOS, MD, DSc
First Department of Orthopaedics, Athens University Medical School, Athens, Greece

ADAM J. PEADEN, DPM
Department of Podiatric Surgery (East Orlando Campus); Department of Medical Education, Florida Hospital East Orlando, Orlando, Florida

CRYSTAL L. RAMANUJAM, DPM
Fellow, Postgraduate Research and Clinical Instructor, Division of Podiatric Medicine and Surgery, Department of Orthopaedic Surgery, The University of Texas Health Science Center at San Antonio, San Antonio, Texas

CHRISTOPHER L. REEVES, DPM, FACFAS
Section Chief, Department of Podiatric Surgery (East Orlando Campus); Attending Physician, Podiatric Medicine and Surgery Residency, Florida Hospital East Orlando; Orlando Foot and Ankle Clinic, Orlando, Florida

DAVID REGULE, MD, PT, MS
Clinical Rheumatologist, Assistant Clinical Professor of Internal medicine, Northeastern Ohio Universities College of Medicine, Rootstown Ohio; Humility of Mary Health Partners, Department of Medical Education, Internal Medicine Teaching Program, Youngstown, Ohio

FRANCINE C. RHINEHART, DPM
PGY-1, PM&S-36, Department of Podiatry, Catholic Health System, Buffalo, New York

BRYAN SAGRAY, DPM
Division of Podiatric Medicine and Surgery, Department of Orthopaedic Surgery, The University of Texas Health science Center at San Antonio, San Antonio, Texas

KAREN SCHORN, MD
Pinehurst Rheumatology Clinic, Southern Pines, North Carolina

AMBER M. SHANE, DPM, FACFAS
Department of Podiatric Surgery (East Orlando Campus); Orlando Foot and Ankle Clinic, Orlando, Florida

HELEN SKOUTELI, MD
Consultant Pediatric Neurologist, Pagkzati, Athens, Greece

JEFFREY SZCZEPANSKI, DPM, FACFAS
Private Practice, Traverse City, Michigan; Diplomate of American Board of Podiatric Surgery, Board Certified in Foot and Reconstructive Rearfoot/Ankle Surgery

JOSEPH R. TREADWELL, DPM, FACFAS
Foot and Ankle Specialists of Connecticut, PC, Danbury, Connecticut

GEORGE TZANOS, MD, DSC
Department of Physical Medicine and Rehabilitation, Thriasio Hospital, Elefsina, Greece

STAMATIOS G. VRETTOS, MS
Pediatric Physical Therapist, Halandri, Athens, Greece

GLEN M. WEINRAUB, DPM, FACFAS
Department of Orthopaedic Surgery, Kaiser Permanente Medical Group, Fremont/Hayward California, Fremont, California; Clinical Assistant Professor, Midwestern University School of Podiatric Medicine, Phoenix, Arizona; Director of GME Kaiser Permanente GSAA, California

ERIKA WOMACK, MS
Research Coordinator, Department of Orthopaedic Surgery, University of Mississippi Medical Center, Jackson, Mississippi

THOMAS ZGONIS, DPM, FACFAS
Director, Podiatric Surgical Residency and Reconstructive Fellowship Programs; Chief, Division of Podiatric Medicine and Surgery; Associate Professor, Department of Orthopedic Surgery, The University of Texas Health Science Center at San Antonio, San Antonio, Texas

CATHERINE ZIMMERMAN, MD
House Officer, Department of Pediatrics, University of Mississippi Medical Center, Jackson, Mississippi

Contents

Dedication   xv

Thomas Zgonis

Foreword   xvii

Thomas Zgonis

Preface: The Pursuit of Surgical Perfection   xix

Lawrence A. Didomenico

Introduction

**An Update on Inflammatory Arthropathies Including Pharmacologic Management
and Preoperative Considerations**   183

David Regule

This article provides an update and overview to the clinical presentations of inflammatory arthropathies. Subtleties to clinical presentations are discussed. Clues are presented which helps the reader arrive at more precise diagnostic labeling. Additionally, pharmacotherapy will be discussed, including precautions in considering the best therapy for the patient with suspected inflammatory, autoimmune, degenerative or neuropathic pain conditions. Finally, preoperative evaluations, management and risks of this patient population are reviewed. Emphasis will be on whether "cardiac clearance" should be requested based on an easy to use algorithm of cardiac risk factors. Finally recommendations based on recent literature of whether immunosuppressants should be withheld preoperatively.

Conservative Treatments for Rheumatoid Arthritis in the Foot and Ankle   193

Joseph M. Anain Jr, Angela R. Bojrab, and Francine C. Rhinehart

Rheumatoid arthritis (RA) is a systemic inflammatory disease that attacks peripheral joints, causing their destruction. Several pharmacologic therapies and physical modalities are available for its treatment. Because of the progressive nature of RA, complementary and alternative medicine therapy in conjunction with conventional medicine is administered to patients with RA. This article discusses the presence of undiagnosed RA in the foot and ankle and reviews the concurrent nonoperative measures in treatment, including pharmacologic and physical modalities.

Medical Imaging and Radiographic Analysis of the Rheumatoid Patient   209

Adam Hicks, Heiko Adams, and Jeffrey Szczepanski

According to the Arthritis Foundation, approximately 1.3 million Americans have rheumatoid arthritis (RA), while an estimated 300,000 children are diagnosed with the disease each year. The disease is 2- to 4-times more common in women than in men and is least common in young men. Current practices in the treatment of RA center on the early detection of the various disease manifestations, specifically joint destruction. The goal of early detection is the implementation of disease-modifying drugs before articular destruction and deformity set in. Advancements in medical imaging have led to methods that facilitate earlier detection and beneficial treatment in the course of RA. Because standard radiographic interpretation assists with diagnosis of later-stage arthritis after articular destruction has occurred, magnetic resonance imaging has proven to be the most effective study for early signs of RA. Other imaging modalities such as ultrasonography and contrast-enhanced computed tomography have also been shown to detect early signs of RA. In conjunction with laboratory testing, these imaging modalities are essential for the early detection and subsequent treatment of RA. Pedal imaging is used by most rheumatologists to detect and monitor disease progression, and by most podiatric surgeons to help direct treatment and plan surgical intervention.

Clinical Manifestations and Treatment of the Pediatric Rheumatoid Patient   219

Lawrence Haber, Erika Womack, Catherine Zimmerman, and Joshua Hughes

The management goal of juvenile rheumatoid arthritis (JRA) is to achieve early diagnosis and treatment so that arthritis can be resolved at an early stage, which avoids long-term damage and provides a good outcome of the affected inflammatory joints. This article describes presentation, classification, evaluation, and treatment of JRA as it relates to the foot and ankle. Because the course of JRA is complex and the optimal management is highly variable in each patient, this article can only offer recommendations. Actual treatment should be individualized to meet the conditions of each patient.

Perioperative Management of the Patient with Rheumatoid Arthritis   235

Allen Mark Jacobs

Familiarity with the systemic manifestations of rheumatoid arthritis as well as familiarity with drug therapy used for the management of rheumatoid arthritis may be helpful in the avoidance of some postoperative complications. Drug effects on soft tissues and bone may complicate reduction, stabilization, and fixation of deformities. Evaluation of the patient with rheumatoid arthritis for extraarticular disease may also explain symptomatology, and reduce the incidence of complications by unrecognized contributions of soft tissue pathology of osseous and articular disorders.

The Surgical Reconstruction of the Rheumatoid Forefoot   243

Alfonso Anthony Haro III, Lacey F. Moore, Karen Schorn,
and Lawrence A. DiDomenico

Rheumatoid arthritis is an autoimmune disorder that presents in females more often than males, and may affect people belonging to any age group. This disease shows no regional or ethnic preference. Although genetic and environmental causes have been proposed, the definitive cause of immunologic susceptibility, as well as viral and bacterial infectious processes that may cause rheumatoid arthritis, have not been identified. This article discusses various reconstructive forefoot surgeries to correct rheumatoid arthritis and the perioperative care of the patients who undergo surgery, along with the radiographic and magnetic resonance imaging findings associated with the disease.

The Surgical Reconstruction of Rheumatoid Midfoot and Hindfoot Deformities   261

Jason D. Neufeld, Glen M. Weinraub, Ernesto S. Hernandez, and Marc S. Co

Dealing with the rheumatoid midfoot and hindfoot is a challenging endeavor. There are numerous perioperative factors that influence surgical outcomes. This article provides a brief overview of the disease process and pertinent details on the surgical management of the rheumatoid midfoot and hindfoot. The pathophysiology, clinical presentation, imaging, conservative treatment options, perioperative management, and surgical intervention for rheumatoid midfoot and hindfoot disease are discussed, with special attention to primary arthrodesis for midfoot and hindfoot reconstruction in the rheumatoid patient, which has been the mainstay of treatment for the last 100 years.

Surgery on the Rheumatoid Ankle Joint: Efficacy Versus Effectiveness   275

Joseph R. Treadwell

This article examines synovectomy and ankle arthrodesis for the rheumatoid ankle joint. Reviews of osteoimmunology and gait analyses specific to rheumatoid arthritis are included. Comparison studies including ankle arthrodesis and total ankle arthroplasty are reviewed.

Total Ankle Arthroplasty in the Rheumatoid Patient   295

Lawrence A. DiDomenico, Joseph R. Treadwell, and Laurence Z. Cain

Total ankle replacement in the rheumatoid patient is a feasible and effective treatment for ankle arthritis. The benefits of ankle prosthesis are good pain relief, acceptable function, and patient satisfaction. It is a joint-sparing procedure for restoring functionality. All investigators of total ankle replacement feel that, as clinicians gain experience with the procedure and related products, difficulties and risks associated with the procedure will decline. Following an early history of failure and poor patient satisfaction, more recent results have shown promise.

The Complications Encountered with the Rheumatoid Surgical Foot and Ankle   313

Christopher L. Reeves, Adam J. Peaden, and Amber M. Shane

Rheumatoid arthritis (RA) is a chronic, degenerative, systemic disease that leads to the destruction of articular cartilage of the joints. Complications, including infection, delays in wound healing, malunion, nonunion, implant failure, and degeneration of adjacent joints soon after primary fusion, have been described in the literature and are generally accepted as commonplace in reconstructive surgeries of the foot and ankle. The combined efforts of the surgeon and supporting physicians to maintain optimal health for the patient, along with the principles discussed in this article, can lead to superior outcomes with fewer complications in the postoperative course.

Current Concepts and Techniques in Foot and Ankle Surgery

Subtalar Joint Arthrodesis, Ankle Arthrodiastasis, and Talar Dome Resurfacing with the Use of a Collagen-Glycosaminoglycan Monolayer   327

Crystal L. Ramanujam, Bryan Sagray, and Thomas Zgonis

Intraarticular fractures of the calcaneus are a common injury to the hindfoot leading to posttraumatic arthrosis of the subtalar joint. Operative treatment with reduction and internal fixation at the time of initial presentation and once the soft tissue envelope is deemed suitable has become the standard of care for the surgical management of calcaneal fractures. However, numerous complications have been associated with calcaneal fractures, most notably subtalar joint arthrosis and calcaneal malunion. The authors describe a method of a delayed subtalar joint arthrodesis, ankle joint arthrodiastasis, and talar resurfacing with positive results for the management of painful posttraumatic concomitant arthrosis of the subtalar and ankle joints.

Selective Percutaneous Myofascial Lengthening of the Lower Extremities in Children with Spastic Cerebral Palsy   335

Evanthia A. Mitsiokapa, Andreas F. Mavrogenis, Helen Skouteli,
Stamatios G. Vrettos, George Tzanos, Anastasios D. Kanellopoulos,
Demetrios S. Korres, and Panayiotis J. Papagelopoulos

Children with spastic cerebral palsy commonly acquire lower extremity musculoskeletal deformities that at some point may need surgical correction. The authors present 58 children with spastic cerebral palsy who underwent selective percutaneous myofascial lengthening of the hip adductor group and the medial or the lateral hamstrings. All the patients were spastic diplegic, hemiplegic, or quadriplegic. The indications for surgery were a primary contracture that interfered with the patients' walking or sitting ability or joint subluxation. Gross motor ability and gross motor function of the children were evaluated using the gross motor function classification system (GMFCS) and the gross motor function measure (GMFM), respectively. The mean time of the surgical procedure was 14 minutes (range, 1 to 27 minutes). All patients were discharged from the hospital setting the same day after the operation. There were no infections, overlengthening, nerve palsies, or vascular complications. Three patients required repeat procedures for relapsed hamstring and adductor contractures at 8, 14, and 16 months postoperatively. At 2 years after the initial operation, all the children improved on their previous functional level; 34 children improved by one GMFCS level, and 5 children improved by two GMFCS levels. The overall improvement in mean GMFM scores was from 71.19 to 83.19.

Index   345

FORTHCOMING ISSUES

July 2010
Heel Pathology
George F. Wallace, DPM, *Guest Editor*

October 2010
Forefoot Pain
D. Martin Chaney, DPM,
and Walter W. Strash, DPM, *Guest Editors*

January 2011
Foot and Ankle Athletic Injuries
Babak Baravarian, DPM, *Guest Editor*

RECENT ISSUES

January 2010
The Pediatric Pes Planovalgus Deformity
Neal M. Blitz, DPM, *Guest Editor*

October 2009
Advances in Wound and Bone Healing
 Adam Landsman, DPM, *Guest Editor*

July 2009
The Importance of the First Ray
Lawrence A. Ford, DPM, *Guest Editor*

RELATED INTEREST

Foot and Ankle Clinics Volume 15, Issue 1 (March 2010)
Traumatic Foot and Ankle Injuries Related to Recent International Conflicts
Edited by Eric Bluman and James Ficke

THE CLINICS ARE NOW AVAILABLE ONLINE!

Access your subscription at:
www.theclinics.com

Dedication

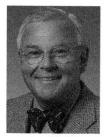

In Memory of Gary Peter Jolly, DPM, FACFAS (1948–2010)

It is with a great sadness that I inform you of the passing of a true pioneer in our podiatric profession. As one of his previous reconstructive fellows and having had the opportunity to join his practice after my fellowship training, I truly believe that he has played a significant role in my academic career. From the first time I saw him in surgery, when I was a student, I realized that my career path was to follow his steps and learn from his tremendous knowledge and experience.

Besides his many professional accomplishments, his kindness, generosity, and honesty will be remembered forever. He was gifted with his teaching and outstanding surgical skills and always curious to test his knowledge in clinical research. He was eager to learn new techniques and ideas and to try something 'outside the box'. He was admired, loved, and honored by all of his family, friends, staff, and colleagues.

He traveled, lectured, and published extensively; performed clinical research; and served as president of the American College of Foot and Ankle Surgeons. He was one of the first podiatric surgeons to start a reconstructive fellowship, because he strongly believed in further education and surgical training. His thinking and surgical procedural approach as well as his exceptional surgical tips and pearls are with me to this day as I try to pass his wisdom to my current trainees. He has taught me so much in two of his most cherished and favorite aspects of foot and ankle surgery: external fixation and plastic reconstruction.

Dr Jolly was also blessed by his family and children. He had a great family environment and his house welcomed friends and guests at all times. He liked the holiday gatherings with family and friends. He was always available to listen and advise anyone who needed his help.

My dearest friend, colleague, and mentor, may God bless you, your family, and all the lives you have touched. Your soul and spirit will be with us forever…

Rest in peace,
The Zgonis Family

Thomas Zgonis, DPM, FACFAS

E-mail address:
zgonis@uthscsa.edu

Clin Podiatr Med Surg 27 (2010) xv
doi:10.1016/j.cpm.2010.02.002
0891-8422/10/$ – see front matter
podiatric.theclinics.com

Foreword: The Rheumatoid Foot and Ankle

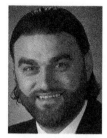

Thomas Zgonis, DPM, FACFAS
Consulting Editor

Rheumatoid arthritis encompasses a wide spectrum of features, from self-limiting disease to a progressively chronic disease with varying degrees of joint destruction commonly affecting the foot and ankle. Surgical reconstruction is becoming more common for treating rheumatoid arthritis, but a simple treatment protocol is not feasible for all patients. In the past, most surgeons were trained with the thought that rheumatoid forefoot deformities were best managed with a panmetatarsal head resection with or without a combined first metatarsophalangeal arthroplasty or arthrodesis, while hindfoot deformities were treated with a triple or pantalar arthrodesis. While these procedures are useful for treating selected rheumatoid patients, they are not always considered for all deformities.

Today, surgeons realize that, to properly select the most appropriate procedures for each patient, the various stages and potential progression of deformities along with the extra-articular manifestations need to be considered in detail. In this issue, the authors selected for this topic have vast knowledge and expertise in this field, making them well qualified to discuss the latest advances in the management of the rheumatoid foot and ankle. Some recent advances have focused on incision planning and surgical exposures to minimize wound-healing complications and the recurrence of deformity. Joint-sparing procedures and ankle implant arthroplasty have become more popular amongst the rheumatoid patient population and have produced reasonably good results. While this topic is rather broad, the authors have done an excellent job in describing these novel techniques while also providing a comprehensive understanding of this chronic inflammatory systemic disease for all physicians treating the rheumatoid foot and ankle.

Thomas Zgonis, DPM, FACFAS
Division of Podiatric Medicine and Surgery
Department of Orthopaedic Surgery
The University of Texas Health Science Center at San Antonio
7703 Floyd Curl Drive–MSC 7776
San Antonio, TX 78229, USA

E-mail address:
zgonis@uthscsa.edu

Clin Podiatr Med Surg 27 (2010) xvii
doi:10.1016/j.cpm.2010.01.003
0891-8422/10/$ – see front matter © 2010 Elsevier Inc. All rights reserved.

Preface

The Pursuit of Surgical Perfection

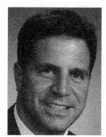

Lawrence A. DiDomenico, DPM, FACFAS
Guest Editor

The "perfect" surgical scenario: You feel good, rested, and confident in the procedure you are about to perform. The patient is in good physical condition, is easy to communicate with, and seems to have a good understanding of what is required postoperatively. After the surgical procedure, you feel like everything worked out perfectly and you are confident that the patient will experience a good outcome.

Then, at the first postoperative visit, or during grand rounds, you review the patient's radiographs and are pleased with the results. Incidentally, you know the patient will most likely be happy with the results as well. But, when you truly evaluate your results with the utmost intellectual honesty, you know there is room for improvement.

This is what I call "the relentless pursuit of surgical perfection," and it is my personal mantra. As surgeons, if we are truthful with ourselves, we should constantly strive to, for example, obtain better reductions, improve fixation placements, and achieve better anatomic alignments in each and every case.

Golf, in a way, is very similar to surgery. Even if you play your best round, once you review your 18 holes, you will most likely find that you had many opportunities to improve your score. The few great shots you had that day leave you with an awesome feeling about your swing and the game. This is what you remember and what drives you to come back the next time to try for even better results.

Practice, as defined by *Encarta Dictionary* (2010): "repeat something to get better; do something as custom." The term relates to what we as surgeons do every day. However, as good as we think we are, or as good as a surgical outcome may be, we should continue to strive for improvement because practicing medicine means that true perfection will always elude us.

Clin Podiatr Med Surg 27 (2010) xix–xx
doi:10.1016/j.cpm.2010.01.002
0891-8422/10/$ – see front matter © 2010 Elsevier Inc. All rights reserved.

podiatric.theclinics.com

I am grateful for the privilege to serve as guest editor for this edition of *Clinics in Podiatric Medicine and Surgery* focusing on rheumatoid arthritis. Foot and ankle surgeons are routinely involved with the management of this disease. In recent years, the management of rheumatoid arthritis both medically and surgically has evolved considerably. The teams of physicians involved with these advances have enhanced the functionality and quality of life for these patients suffering from rheumatoid arthritis. The objective of this issue of *Clinics in Podiatric Medicine and Surgery* is to introduce readers to the most recent advances in medical and surgical management of rheumatoid arthritis of the foot and ankle from selected physicians with relevant expertise.

My wish is that this issue will encourage and enable surgeons to provide improved care for patients afflicted with this unfortunate and disabling disease.

I would like to thank Dr Thomas Zgonis for providing me the opportunity to serve as guest editor for this issue. Additionally, I would like to thank my family, as well as the families of all the contributing writers, for their support, which has enabled us to create what we hope is a valuable and lasting medical resource.

Lawrence A. DiDomenico, DPM, FACFAS
Reconstructive Rearfoot & Ankle Surgical Fellowship
Ankle and Foot Care Centers
Ohio College of Podiatric Medicine
8175 Market Street, Youngstown
OH 44512, USA

E-mail address:
LD5353@aol.com

An Update on Inflammatory Arthropathies Including Pharmacologic Management and Preoperative Considerations

David Regule, MD, PT, MS[a,b,]*

KEYWORDS

- Inflammatory arthropathy • Erosive conditions
- Pharmacotherapy • Surgical Risks

Important issues for any physician and surgeon to be aware of during the perioperative period of their rheumatoid patients include pharmacology concerns, and other screening questions and procedures prior to surgery. This article introduces the workup for possible rheumatoid arthritis in patients who are suspected of having underlying connective tissue disease, but are not currently seeing a rheumatologist. Acute flares of inflammatory arthritis, such as gouty arthropathy, cellulitis, rheumatoid arthritis, inflammatory bowel disease associated arthropathy, psoriatic arthropathy, or reactive arthritis after a recent viral infection can be difficult to differentiate. Finally, this article also discusses the pharmacologic management of inflammatory arthritis and gout.

DIFFERENTIAL DIAGNOSIS OF SUSPECTED INFLAMMATORY OR EROSIVE CONDITIONS OF THE FEET

If signs and symptoms of inflammatory arthritis with warm, tender, swollen joints, such as an inflamed first metatarsophalangeal joint (MTPJ), are noted on examination, then

[a] Department of Internal Medicine, Northeastern Ohio Universities College of Medicine, 4209 State Route 44, Rootstown, OH 44272, USA
[b] Humility of Mary Health Partners, Department of Medical Education, Internal Medicine Teaching Program, 1044 Belmont Avenue, Youngstown, OH 44501, USA
* Humility of Mary Health Partners, Department of Medical Education, Internal Medicine Teaching Program, 1044 Belmont Avenue, Youngstown, OH 44501.
E-mail address: dregule@yahoo.com

Clin Podiatr Med Surg 27 (2010) 183–191
doi:10.1016/j.cpm.2009.12.010
0891-8422/10/$ – see front matter © 2010 Elsevier Inc. All rights reserved.

podiatric.theclinics.com

important historical clues should be sought to help differentiate possible causes. If the related cause is secondary to trauma, then hemarthrosis and soft tissue swelling related to the traumatic injury is likely to be noted. If this swollen joint occurred insidiously without trauma, septic arthritis or cellulitis should be considered. Did the patient describe a prior paronychial infection that then spread into the length of the great toe? Was there a preceding break in the skin that would lead into a deeper infection or cellulitis? Frequently, bacterial cellulitis in the feet is preceded by breaks in the skin from edematous feet with tinea pedis infections between the toes. A break in the skin over a swollen joint or any new pain around a previous arthroplasty would be strongly suspicious for septic arthritis. Appropriate workup for this includes complete blood count, needle aspiration of synovial fluid through a nonerythematous skin, and appropriate medical imaging.

A history of recurring swollen, tender, first MTPJ synovitis raises strong suspicion for gouty arthropathy. Chronic but waxing and waning forefoot synovitis with morning stiffness, and pain with ambulation in the forefoot like "walking on marbles" could suggest rheumatoid arthritis. This condition would differ from the plantar fasciitis "sharp" heel/arch pain with the first few steps in the morning. Acute onset of less than a few weeks of migratory arthritis plus a history of nonspecific erythematous rash could suggest a postviral reactive arthritis or a drug-induced lupus-like syndrome. The clinician should ask about preceding infections in the past few weeks or new medications the patients may have taken, such as antibiotics or hydralazine. Malar rash of the face, diffuse rashes, or photosensitivity (rash or sickness after being in the sun, excluding heat exhaustion) in association with fevers, polyarthritis, and serositis (complaints of pain with breathing) could be systemic lupus or a drug-induced lupus-like picture. Ankle and knee swelling associated with simultaneous fevers, diarrhea, and weight loss could signify arthritis associated with inflammatory bowel disease.

Several associations should be looked for on physical examination to help clarify the diagnosis. Bilateral second to fourth MTPJ synovitis with metacarpophalangeal joint (MCPJ) synovitis or tenderness of the hands and wrists suggests rheumatoid arthritis. Ankle synovitis can be seen with sarcoidosis in conjunction with erythema nodosum (purple spots) on the anterior tibia. A chest radiograph would be diagnostic of sarcoidosis if hilar adenopathy is noted. Disseminated *Neisseria* gonococcal infection may have preceding rash, pustula lesions, and tenosynovitis. Psoriatic plaques and nail pitting may show a sausage digit swelling of dactylitis in psoriatic arthritis. The finding of nail pitting should be present to suggest inflammatory arthritis associated with psoriasis. The nail pitting or periungual swelling and changes that would suggest a connective tissue disease might be more specific when looking at the hands, which would exclude the onychomycosis present in the feet, whereas dactylitis is more obvious when looking at the toes.

On physical examination a few features are diagnostic. Although not specific, the author recommends the squeeze test of both hands MCPJs (like performing a hand shake) and both forefeet MTPJs to screen for rheumatoid arthritis. This area is where pain is reproduced in the middle of the foot (second to fourth MTPJ) when squeezing, with no tenderness over the medial or lateral edges of forefoot where painful calluses may be located.

Rheumatoid nodules on the fingers or distal to the olecranon on the forearm may support rheumatoid arthritis diagnosis. Gouty tophi behind the olecranon posterior to the elbows or located in the toes, fingers, or along the ear auricle support a gouty arthritis diagnosis. Large nodules over distal phalangeal joints of the hands likely means generalized hypertrophic degenerative joint disease that can have mild inflammation and can be erosive. Dactylitis and nail pitting plus psoriatic plaques support a diagnosis of psoriatic arthropathy.

Severe decreased lumbar flexion range of motion and Achilles tendonitis, with a history of chronic inflammatory sacroiliac stiffness and pain in morning for more than 30 minutes improved by exercise, could mean ankylosing spondylitis. Periungual erythema can be present in some connective tissue diseases such as lupus. Clubbing of the nail bed and pain that is aggravated when the limb is in a gravity-dependent position and relieved when elevated should prompt a pulmonary evaluation for hypertrophic pulmonary osteoarthropathy.

Loose hypermobile joints and an overpronated foot may suggest generalized ligamentous laxity syndrome. A positive tender point survey can be performed by asking the patients if they feel tenderness with enough mild pressure to blanch one's thumb when pushing over multiple areas of the body. A positive response over skin, bone, muscle, and joints might suggest anxiety or other causes of allodynia, such as reflex sympathetic dystrophy or a fibromyalgia, but not inflammatory arthritis. To screen for this, slight pressure is placed on the tibias, forearms, and anterior chest; if these areas are tender or "feel bruised" then the patient likely suffers from a systemic neuropathic processing disorder such as fibromyalgia. Shooting, lancinating pains, and numb feelings particularly in the toes are more highly suggestive of neuropathic pain, and appropriate diagnostic testing, such as monofilament sensory testing, and ruling out peripheral arterial disease should be done.

If erosive changes are noted on plain radiographs of the feet, a foot and ankle specialist should consider nodular familial erosive osteoarthritis and posttraumatic osteoarthritis. However, connective tissue diseases with a history of inflammation, such as rheumatoid arthritis or erosive gouty arthropathy, should be considered. Radiographs of rheumatoid arthritis may show classic changes of marginal erosions, periarticular osteopenia, and possibly soft tissue swelling. The first MTPJ classically shows erosive changes with long-standing uncontrolled gout (in addition, crystal layering may be seen on musculoskeletal ultrasound examination). Psoriatic arthropathy tends to cause hypertrophic and erosive changes on radiographs, similar to familial erosive osteoarthritis. Other connective tissue diseases such as lupus do not tend to cause erosive changes. Postosteomyelitis erosive changes, particularly in diabetic patients, can be a consideration. Charcot foot changes secondary to long-standing neuropathy can easily be confused with late-stage rheumatoid erosive deformities on radiographs. Clinical correlation or a formal radiologist interpretation of these films could assist in distinguishing these conditions.

If an inflammatory condition such as rheumatoid arthritis is suspected, synovitis of the forefoot or ankle is noted. A trial of prednisone, 20 mg daily for 7 days, if helpful, possibly could support a diagnosis of inflammatory arthritis. The author recommends obtaining blood work, checking for rheumatoid factor, and that anticyclic citrullinated peptide be drawn to screen for rheumatoid factor. If no infection is present, inflammatory markers such as erythrocyte sedimentation rate and nonsensitive C-reactive proteins (CRPs) can be helpful (frequently the laboratory will draw a high-/ultrasensitive CRP that is only helpful in cardiac coronary artery disease risk stratification). An antinuclear antibody usually is not helpful unless rashes, photosensitivity, serositis, fever, or other symptoms are noted. A radiograph may help rule out a stress fracture or other causes. If erosive changes are noted on the radiograph, an antinuclear antibody test is not needed, because other autoimmune or connective tissue diseases, such as lupus, do not cause erosive changes.

In addition, a uric acid (UA) level of 4 to 10 mmol/L may not be helpful in diagnosing acute gout. UA levels are routinely artificially suppressed during acute flares and are not accurate. A UA level less than 4 mmol/L, however, makes gouty arthropathy flare less likely. A UA level greater than 10 mmol/L means that the patient is at high risk for developing gouty arthropathy at some point in the future, but may not necessarily mean that current symptoms are due to gout. Furthermore, if there seems to be a classic history of an episode at the first MTPJ with pain, swelling, redness and, most importantly, severe tenderness and good response to cold therapy, then one can make a presumptive diagnosis of likely gout. Note that a definite diagnosis of gouty arthropathy can only be made by polarized microscope visualization of urate crystals seen intracellularly in neutrophils from affected synovial fluid, with inflammatory fluid more than 5000 cells/mL^3, normal white blood cell count, and negative cultures. However, a fairly certain diagnosis can also be made if the physical examination yields tophus changes or if the musculoskeletal ultrasound of affected joints yields classic layering of crystals. Erosive changes in the margins of the head of the first metatarsal are also a classic sign of gouty arthropathy.

PHARMACOLOGY

If a systemic inflammatory condition is suspected, nonsteroidal anti-inflammatory drugs (NSAIDs) or a short course of prednisone can be initiated. If used during the short term at low doses, then risks with these medications may be minimized; however, the following paragraphs review some of the risks associated with the use of these medications.

All NSAIDs have concerns for acute and chronic renal insufficiency, salt retention, volume overload, and blood pressure increase, especially in patients with liver cirrhosis, renal failure, or congestive heart failure. Myocardial infarction is a known rare complication of any NSAIDs and not just COX-2 inhibitors, such as rofecoxib (Vioxx) or valdecoxib (Bextra). Risks and benefits need to be considered in those with risk factors for coronary artery disease. Most significant risk factors include long-standing diabetes or a history of prior myocardial infarction. Less significant risk factors include uncontrolled hypertension, current tobacco use, untreated high cholesterol, or early myocardial infarction in a first-degree family member (in father before the age of 55 years or in mother before the age of 65 years). If the patient had a recent (<6 months ago) myocardial infarction or cerebrovascular accident, this author would recommend against NSAID therapy.

If a patient is on a daily low-dose "baby" aspirin for cardiac prophylaxis, ibuprofen has been shown to block the effects of the platelet inhibition from aspirin. Therefore, part of the risk of taking chronic NSAIDs is increased possibility of coronary artery disease events because of the protective effects of aspirin being blocked. Options include taking the aspirin and then waiting 1 to 2 hours before taking the NSAIDs. Celecoxib (Celebrex), a COX-2 inhibitor, can be taken at the same time as the aspirin without this interaction. Alternatively, once-a-day inexpensive medications such as generic meloxicam (Mobic, which is COX-2 predominant) can be taken in the evening and aspirin in the morning; this has been shown to have little interaction. Data support the conclusion that COX-2 inhibitors are preferable to nonselective NSAIDs in patients with chronic pain and cardiovascular risk needing low-dose aspirin, but relative risks and benefits should be assessed individually for each patient.

Peptic ulcer and erosive gastropathy, particularly in the elderly, is a known complication of chronic NSAID therapy. Life-threatening gastrointestinal bleeding can occur, particularly in those patients who are also on Coumadin, even in the absence of preceding abdominal pain. If chronic NSAID therapy is being considered in the elderly or patients with prior gastric bleeding ulcer, prophylactic proton pump inhibitor (PPI) therapy (such as esomeprazole [Nexium], lansoprazole [Prevacid], omeprazole [Prilosec]) should also be given concurrently to reduce the risk of gastrointestinal erosions or ulcerations. COX-2 specific inhibitors such as celecoxib (Celebrex) and possibly meloxicam (Mobic) have been shown to be safer regarding gastrointestinal bleeding risks.

Chronic use of steroids is well known to cause multiple complications, particularly when used in high doses. In the acute situation, the patient should be warned of extra energy, possible irritability, and sleep difficulty. Steroids could also cause a flare of a manic episode. Low dosage or possible avoidance of steroids in patients with bipolar disorder or history of manic episodes in the past is highly recommended. Diabetic patients should also be warned of an increase in blood sugar levels. Hypertensive patients should be advised of possible blood pressure increase or salt/fluid retention. All patients should be advised of increased appetite and potential for weight gain if they are on steroid therapy long term.

In addition, chronic use of steroids should be avoided and alternative medications should be attempted to limit the dose and length of steroid therapy. However, if chronic steroids, more than 5 mg prednisone for more than 3 months, are to be prescribed, then a few precautions should be taken. First, bone protection medications should be started to counter the deleterious effects of steroids on bone mass. One calcium capsule (1200 mg total per day) with a meal twice daily increases absorption in those patients also on PPI therapy. The patients are also encouraged to take at least 1000 units of vitamin D, once per day. Even if patients have a normal bone density on dual energy x-ray absorptiometry (DEXA) scan, initiation of bisphosphonate therapy, such as risedronate (Actonel), alendronate (Fosamax), or ibandronate (Boniva), is warranted for patients who are not likely to get pregnant and are on chronic steroids. Once chronic steroid therapy is started, fracture risk increases before a detectable loss of bone on DEXA scan is noted. If the steroid is later stopped, then the concomitant bisphosphonate therapy can be stopped. Next, the patient should be advised to "stress dose" his or her steroids during periods of significant illness or surgery, and not abruptly stop taking chronic steroids because of the risk of acquired adrenal insufficiency. Lastly, the risk of stomach ulcerations usually only occurs in chronic steroid users who are also concurrently on NSAIDs and therefore, only these patients require prophylactic PPI therapy.

The use of disease-modifying antirheumatic drugs (DMARDs) in rheumatoid arthritic patients is not discussed in depth here, because these are most likely used by practitioners such as rheumatologists. This article addresses perioperative concerns related to these medications. The author highly recommends physicians and surgeons to observe for ongoing breakthrough active inflammation in the MTPJs in rheumatoid arthritic patients and report this to the rheumatologist for intensification of therapy. If a fragility fracture occurs (nontraumatic or minimally traumatic fracture after a fall from a standing height), then the primary care physician or rheumatologist should be advised as to initiation of possible chronic bisphosphonate therapy or temporary use of calcitonin nasal spray within a few weeks of the fracture, and the patient should be considered to be at a high risk for future fractures. With deep soft tissue infections or cellulitis, the patient with rheumatoid arthritis on tumor necrosis factor (TNF) inhibitor blockade (etanercept [Enbrel], adalimumab [Humira], infliximab [Remicade]) should be advised to delay taking their next dose until after the infection has cleared or significantly improved, and no fever noted.

The surgeon may observe an unusual or rare complication of DMARD therapy. A new peripheral neuropathy is known to occur in leflunomide (Arava). Flare congestive heart failure with worsening lower extremity edema or multiple sclerosis, such as a demyelinating condition with new upward Babinski, can rarely occur after initiation of TNF inhibitor blockade. Finally, intravenous (IV) bisphosphonate therapy should be considered for patients with chronic neuropathy and hyperemic/warm feet that may be undergoing Charcot changes because the bones begin to collapse and degenerate.

GOUT MANAGEMENT

If an acute flare of gout is suspected, NSAIDs or steroids are recommended. If the patient has experienced a recent myocardial infarction or known moderate renal insufficiency, the use of NSAIDs is not recommended. The author does not recommend high doses of colchicine because of the frequency of diarrhea and gastrointestinal distress with doses above 2 to 3 tablets given in a 24-hour period. During an acute flare, any NSAID can be used; however, typically indomethacin, 50 mg every 8 hours for a few doses, is usually prescribed. If the patient is hospitalized or is seen in the emergency room, 30 mg of ketorolac (Toradol), IV can be given to obtain relief. Prednisone, 20 to 40 mg daily to be tapered over 10 to 20 days, can be initiated. If only one joint is involved and a low index of suspicion for infection is noticed, then aspiration and injection of steroid can be performed.

If a patient has had multiple recurring gouty attacks, tophi or erosive changes are noted and a long-term prophylactic therapy is started. As the acute flare subsides, the author uses a bridge therapy of colchicine, 0.6 mg every day to twice per day, for prophylaxis for 3 to 6 months while more definitive urate-lowering therapy such as allopurinol is usually being titrated upward. Approximately 1 to 2 weeks after the acute flare, the author would then start allopurinol, 100 mg daily, while titration up to 600 mg daily of allopurinol can be done slowly over months. It is suggested that this should be increased by 100 mg every 3 to 4 weeks and UA levels monitored to achieve a goal of greater than 6.0. Patients need to be advised that when allopurinol is initiated or stopped it can provoke a flare; therefore, gouty flares may worsen when initiating chronic UA-lowering therapy. Allopurinol should not be stopped if a patient has chronically been taking it or if a break through acute gouty attack occurs, because this may prolong the flare.

If a severe rash occurs when starting allopurinol, this may be a sign of a severe life-threatening Stevens-Johnson skin reaction. If a rash is noted, the patient is recommended to discontinue the allopurinol immediately. Other UA-lowering medications can also be used. However, allopurinol is frequently a first-line agent. Losartan (Cozaar) and fenofibrate (Tricor), besides their primary action as blood pressure–lowering and triglyceride-lowering medications, respectively, also help lower UA. Allopurinol (a xanthine oxidase inhibitor) helps overproducers and underexcretors of UA. Probenecid only helps when patients are not excreting enough UA, and UA therefore accumulates in the tissue. A 24-hour urine collection for UA that is low (<400 mmol/L) supports probenecid or allopurinol use being helpful. However, high UA in the urine (>800 mmol/L), history of UA kidney stones, chronic renal insufficiency, and multiple drug interactions make probenecid a less attractive alternative. Finally, a new agent, feboxustat (Uloric), available as 40-mg and 80-mg once-daily dosing, is a more powerful alternative to allopurinol or can be used for those with allopurinol intolerance. Cost of this drug, however, is a limiting factor.

PREOPERATIVE EVALUATION

Diabetes mellitus, hypertension, and asthma should be well controlled prior to surgery. For example, blood pressure greater than 180/100 mm Hg or blood sugar level greater than 300 mg/dL should be addressed before surgery. Active wheezing in a patient using a rescue albuterol inhaler more than twice a day should delay surgery until pulmonary stabilization. If the patient has chronic lung disease and requires chronic home oxygen or pulse oximetry less than 90%, then pulmonary consultation might be prudent before surgery.

Screening question to be asked before surgery might uncover some perioperative risks. Allergies to anesthetics or complications with prior surgeries, such as excessive bleeding, could alert one to potential complications and possibly modify perioperative evaluation. Preoperative blood work is not usually needed in the young patient. The author would ask if there is an incidence of recurring nosebleeds or if the patient is on coumadin therapy; then preoperative prothrombin time and activated partial thromboplastin time could be assessed. However, if the patient previously had teeth pulled, a surgical procedure, or suturing of a wound without excessive bleeding, then the risk for an undiagnosed congenital bleeding diasthesis would be exceedingly rare, so preoperative prothrombin time and activated partial thromboplastin time is not recommended. The patient must be asked about chronic diuretic use when he or she has low potassium or renal insufficiency, and screening blood work, if not recently done, should be carried out.

Specifically, the rheumatologic patient has 2 concerns that need to be addressed. The patient should be asked about chronic steroid use greater than 5 mg for more than 3 months in the past year; if the answer is yes, then stress dose steroids should be used for 4 days in the perioperative period for moderately involved orthopedic procedures such as ankle arthrodesis. Typically 20 mg/d of IV or oral equivalent methylprednisone (or 25 mg prednisone) administered on the day of surgery and tapered for the next 1 to 2 days, then discontinued or returned to baseline prednisone equivalent dose should help to augment the adrenal insufficient patient. All patients with chronic long-standing rheumatoid arthritis or ankylosing spondylitis who are about to undergo surgery involving endotracheal intubation of the airway should have screening preoperative cervical spine radiograph with open-mouth views to assess for the risk of atlanto-axial laxity and compression of the upper cervical cord during intubation.

A further screening question worth asking is whether excessive snoring or gasping occurs while the patient is sleeping. Usually this information is best obtained by asking the patient's partner. Furthermore, if the patient has a neck circumference greater than 17 in (43 cm) then he or she could be at risk for obstructive sleep apnea (OSA). An undiagnosed mild case of OSA might decompensate the night after surgery if recent benzodiazepines or anesthetics during the operative period relax the muscles of the throat region, leading to more severe obstruction. Worsening OSA could then lead to desaturation and increased risk of sudden cardiac arrhythmias. The patient's history of excessive snoring and neck size greater than 17 in might benefit with overnight continuous pulse oximetry or preventative continuous positive airway pressure the night after surgery.

However, of most concern to the surgeon should be identifying those patients who would be at a greatest risk for cardiac death in the perioperative period. The American College of Cardiology (ACC) and the American Heart Association (AHA) have developed guidelines for preoperative cardiac risk stratification, which were revised in 2007. For any emergent surgery, this assessment does not apply because the need for surgery may outweigh the possible risk of cardiac death related to the surgery.

Types of surgeries are categorized by risks and graded as vascular, intermediate, or low.

1. Superficial procedure and most ambulatory surgery is graded as low-risk surgery with cardiac risk usually less than 1%, and these low-risk procedures do not require preoperative cardiac assessment.
2. Orthopedic surgery (such as an ankle arthrodesis) would come under intermediate-risk procedure, with cardiac risk generally 1% to 5%. Most of these patients do not

require cardiac evaluation; however, some follow-up questions should be asked about the patient before surgery. Electrocardiograms are not necessary in those surgical candidates younger than 35 years. Electrocardiogram can be obtained in patients older than 50 years or those with diabetes, peripheral vascular disease, hypertension, high cholesterol, in current smokers, and in those with family history of heart attack (in father before the age of 55 years or in mother before 65 years).

3. Most major vascular procedures, excluding minor procedures such as carotid endarterectomies, are considered the highest-risk surgeries and most require more formal cardiac evaluation, including cardiac stress testing.

The next consideration after the type of surgery would be whether the patient has an active cardiac issue such that the stress of surgery might lead to acute decompensation. Recent myocardial infarction should require cardiology clearance. Patients who have undergone recent angioplasty with stenting should not have aspirin and clopidogrel bisulfate (Plavix) discontinued during the perioperative period. Drug-eluting stents require 1 year of aspirin and Plavix, whereas nondrug-eluting coronary stenting requires only 3 months of consistent dual therapy after the stent is placed.

Otherwise, asking questions and auscultating heart and lungs will detect active cardiac issues that might first need to be addressed. Screening for unstable coronary angina is done by asking about exertional chest pain or pressure with activity. The patient must be asked about progressive shortness of breath when lying down at night, or bipedal edema or basilar crackles on examination, which are signs of possible decompensated heart failure. New atrial fibrillation that is not ventricular-rate controlled (irregular, irregular rhythm with rate >100 on examination) should be addressed before surgery. Severe valvular disease would be screened by auscultating for louder than 3/6 systolic murmurs or any diastolic murmurs. A 3/6 or softer systolic murmur does not require echocardiography or further evaluation.

For patients without any active cardiac conditions, planned low-risk surgery can proceed without any further evaluation. For higher-risk surgeries like most complex orthopedic procedures, functional capacity is next evaluated. Only those who have low functional capacity are considered to be at-risk patients. Metabolic equivalents (METs) range from 1 to more than 10. Surgical candidates who score less than 4 METs require further questioning. However, being able to climb a flight of stairs or walk up a hill without resting roughly estimates the ability to perform 4 METs. Thus, if patients can achieve this without difficulty they are "cleared" and considered at low cardiac risk. If METs are low or unknown because the patient cannot climb stairs because of lung disease or feet/ankle pain, then further questioning is required.

If the moderate-risk orthopedic surgical candidate with MET less than 4 is younger than 50 years old, no other cardiac screening other than electrocardiography is required if he or she has no active cardiac conditions as mentioned earlier. However, if the moderate-risk surgical candidate is older than 50 years and cannot climb one flight of steps without dyspnea, then assessment of cardiac status, including a stress test, is recommended if he or she has multiple high-risk medical illnesses and 2 or more of the following 5 conditions: previous history of heart attack/ischemic heart disease, compensated or previous heart failure, cerebrovascular disease, renal insufficiency with creatinine level more than 2, and insulin requiring long standing diabetic. Perioperative β-blockade or noninvasive stress testing may be required on patients with 2 or more of the aforementioned clinical risk factors. These patients should be referred to a cardiologist or a primary care physician prior to moderate-risk surgery.

The algorithm mentioned earlier by the ACC/AHA 2007 guidelines sounds complicated, but it actually has been simplified from previous guidelines with some easy screening questions so that low-risk patients can be easily identified and surgery may be scheduled without necessarily sending the patient for medical or cardiac clearance. To complete the review, it is necessary to determine if emergent surgery is required and then proceed as soon as possible. If low-risk ambulatory surgery is involved, no cardiac screening is required. For higher-risk vascular procedures, cardiac screening should be done. For intermediate surgical procedures such as fracture repair, a few questions should be asked. The patients should also be asked about recent myocardial infarction or coronary stenting. They must also be questioned about anginal chest pain or orthopnea, which could mean congestive heart failure exacerbation or coronary artery disease. On examination, irregular rhythms or known atrial fibrillation with current rate higher than 100, basilar crackles in the bases of both lungs, or loudness of systolic murmur more than 3/6 requires further evaluation. Next, the patients are asked if they can negotiate a flight of stairs without resting or if their age is less than 50 years; if so then these patients do not require further cardiac assessment other than perhaps an electrocardiogram. Only those older than 50 years and with MET less than 4, and undergoing a moderate-risk surgery with 2 or more of the following prior medical problems, namely coronary artery disease, cerebral vascular accident, congestive heart failure, moderate renal disease, and long-standing insulin, require medical clearance or assessment of cardiac risk, and possibly a stress test or initiation of perioperative β-blocker drug.

Conservative Treatments for Rheumatoid Arthritis in the Foot and Ankle

Joseph M. Anain Jr, DPM[a,b,*], Angela R. Bojrab, DPM[c],
Francine C. Rhinehart, DPM[c]

KEYWORDS

• Rheumatoid arthritis • Gait • Physical therapy • Foot and ankle

Rheumatoid arthritis (RA) is a systemic inflammatory disease that attacks peripheral joints, causing their destruction. The cause of RA is still yet undetermined. However, studies have suggested the disease to be linked to viral infection, directly or indirectly triggering the immune response of class II major histocompatibility complex and specifically human leukocyte antigen DR4.[1] This response concludes in the final cascade release of degradative enzymes and proteases, causing joint destruction that leads to pain, immobility, and foot malformations.[1]

The prevalence of RA worldwide is 1%, with women having twice the affinity than men and age ranging from 45 to 65 years.[2,3] Clinically, patients with RA initially present with foot pain, and foot and ankle specialists may be the first physicians who encounter the patient and have the opportunity to diagnose, treat, and make appropriate referrals. According to Aronow and Hakim-Zargar,[4] 89% of 1000 patients afflicted with RA had feet involvement; 66.9% were affected in the hindfoot, and 8.8% in the ankle. The time of onset and duration of the disease directly correlates with more proximal involvement of the joints in the foot. RA is a progressive disease, causing pain, fatigue, disabling foot deformities, antalgic gait, a decrease in the activities of daily living (ADLs), and other psychosocial problems. Oldfield and Felson,[2] in an evidence-based review, noted the progressive-destructive nature of RA and its effects on patients' ADLs. They found that 92% of patients with RA have foot abnormalities that are painful, causing their gait pattern to become antalgic and slow

[a] Department of Podiatry, Catholic Health System, Sisters Hospital, 2157 Main Street, Buffalo, NY 14214, USA
[b] Podiatric Medical Education, Catholic Health System, 2157 Main Street, Buffalo, NY 14214, USA
[c] Department of Podiatry, Catholic Health System, 2157 Main Street, Buffalo, NY 14214, USA
* Corresponding author. Department of Podiatry, Catholic Health System, Sisters Hospital, 2157 Main Street, Buffalo, NY 14214.
E-mail address: JMANAIN@aol.com

Clin Podiatr Med Surg 27 (2010) 193–207
doi:10.1016/j.cpm.2009.12.003
0891-8422/10/$ – see front matter © 2010 Elsevier Inc. All rights reserved.

podiatric.theclinics.com

shuffling. This disease along with its local destructive effects on peripheral joints can cause significant disability, which could affect the patient's ADLs. About 55% of patients who had RA for 2 years had difficulties in performing simple ADLs, such as household chores, recreational activities, and other leisure activities, whereas 30% of patients, within 3 years of the disease process, had excessive limitations in ADLs and quit their jobs, assuming RA-associated disability.[2]

This article discusses how to recognize the presentation of RA, if not already diagnosed, and reviews the concurrent nonoperative measures in treatment, including pharmacologic and physical modalities. Pharmacologic therapy is an important aspect of the treatment for patients with RA. Several therapies are available for use in patients with this condition, which include the use of nonsteroidal antiinflammatory drugs (NSAIDs), disease-modifying antirheumatic drugs (DMARDs), glucocorticoids, and analgesics. For many patients, these medications are given either individually or in combination.[1] Nonpharmacologic treatment modalities include joint protection programs, electrophysical modalities, exercise and physical activities, and dietary/ herbal therapies. It is also necessary to make appropriate referrals to a multidisciplinary team of physical and occupational therapists to help further manage the disease. Because of the progressive nature of RA, it is apt for patients to try other treatment options. One such option is the complementary and alternative medicine (CAM) therapy in conjunction with conventional medicine. Complementary medicine covers a broad range of homeopathic medicines, ranging from dietary supplements, such as herbs and vitamins, to movement therapies, such as tai chi, and even acupuncture.[3]

PHARMACOLOGIC THERAPIES
Analgesics

Topical medications such as capsaicin or diclofenac and oral medications such as acetaminophen and tramadol may be used to alleviate pain associated with RA to a small extent. These therapies do not help prevent the disease progress, they only help to alleviate some of the pain. The advantage of these analgesics, in comparison to non-steroidal antiinflammatories, is their ability to spare the gastric mucosa from ulceration. They may, however, cause or aggrevate existing constipation, renal or hepatic impairment.

NSAIDs

One of the most common treatments of RA is the administration of NSAIDs. NSAIDs inhibit cyclooxygenase (COX) enzymes and thus decrease the production of prostaglandins.[5] Prostaglandins serve as a protective layer of the mucous membrane found in the stomach lining. Sometimes combinations of NSAIDs and drugs that protect the mucous membranes can help reduce the occurrence of ulcerations. Selective COX-2 inhibitors, called coxibs, seem to have efficacy comparable to nonselective NSAIDs and are less likely to cause gastrointestinal (GI) toxicity. However, they are not less likely to cause renal toxicity. Some nonselective NSAIDs currently being used include diclofenac, ketoprofen, nabumetone, naproxen, and sulindac. Some selective COX-2 inhibitors include celecoxib and meloxicam.[6] The risk of gastroduodenal damage, renal disease, or heart failure should be assessed before prescribing NSAIDs because these medications have the potential to cause serious problems. NSAIDs may reversibly inhibit platelet function and prolong bleeding time.[7]

Several coxibs have been removed from the market as a result of their dangerous side effects. Rofecoxib was taken off the market because of the chance of increased risk of myocardial infarction and strokes in many patients. Valdecoxib was removed from the market because of cardiovascular and dermatologic side effects.[8] Treatment guidelines from The Medical Letter show that naproxen was the NSAID that was associated with the highest risk of bleeding. If the NSAID was given in conjunction with low-dose aspirin, then the risk increased even higher. According to treatment guidelines from The Medical Letter, diclofenac and ibuprofen have the lowest risk associated with upper GI bleeding.[5]

DMARDs

DMARDs have the potential to reduce or prevent joint damage and preserve joint integrity and function, if used early and aggressively enough in the treatment of RA. They are also used for other arthritic diseases such as lupus, psoriatic arthritis, and ankylosing spondylitis. It may take anywhere from 1 to 6 months for this type of therapy to become effective in a patient.[9] There are 2 types of DMARDs, nonbiologic and biologic. Nonbiologic DMARDs have a much slower onset and require regular monitoring for side effects. Nonbiologic DMARDs include methotrexate, hydroxychloroquine, and sulfasalazine. Biologic DMARDs generally target cytokines and typically include interleukin-1 receptor antagonists.[5] Many patients receive a combination of an NSAID and at least one DMARD, and at times they are combined with a low-dose oral glucocorticoid. If disease remission is observed, regular NSAID or glucocorticoid treatment may no longer be needed.[10]

DMARDs do not cure arthritis, they only help control it. For this reason, if remission or optimal control is achieved with DMARD therapy, it often is continued at a maintenance dosage. Discontinuing the DMARD may reactivate the disease process.

There are several side effects that are associated with DMARDs. Hydroxychloroquine may cause retinal damage. Although this is a rare side effect, it should be taken into consideration. If caught early enough, the retinal toxicity may be reversible.[5] Sulfasalazine may create hematologic toxicities such as leukopenia. It is recommended that liver enzyme levels be tested before prescribing sulfasalazine to a patient and the test be repeated throughout the treatment process.[5] DMARDS can also affect the immune system and consequently can make the patient more prone to infections. Some can cause birth defects if taken by women who are pregnant or may become pregnant.[10]

Methotrexate (MTX) is typically one of the first-line DMARDs often used by clinicians. MTX is a structural analog of folic acid that can competitively inhibit the binding of dihydrofolic acid (FH2) to the enzyme dihydrofolate reductase (DHFR). DHFR is responsible for reducing FH2 to folinic acid (FH4), which is the active intracellular metabolite. Thus, MTX decreases the amount of intracellular FH4 available and affects the metabolic pathways within the cell that are FH4-dependent. These pathways include purine and pyrimidine metabolism and amino acid and polyamine synthesis.[11] In several studies, MTX showed significant improvements in the peripheral joints. MTX has rare toxicities such as hepatic fibrosis and cirrhosis.[5]

Researchers now have new information regarding what could cause the development and progression of periarticular autoimmune diseases: proinflammatory cytokine interleukin (IL) 6. One of the newer treatments that is being tried in combination with DMARDs is tocilizumab. Tocilizumab is humanized anti–IL-6 receptor monoclonal antibody. It has been approved for use only in Japan. In the United States it is still under the trial phase. This drug acts by binding to IL-6 and interfering with the signal transmission, leading to reductions in the inflammatory mediator production. There are several side effects that are associated with this newer treatment, which include liver function abnormalities, hyperlipidemia, and neutropenia. Tocilizumab has shown promising effects; and there is a greater success rate in controlling RA when this drug is used in combination with other DMARDs. It is important to remember that only a rheumatologist or a physician with expertise in treating RA should prescribe DMARDs because of the serious side effects and high costs associated with this therapy.[12,13]

Glucocorticoids

One of the most controversial treatments of RA is the use of glucocorticoids. They exhibit antiinflammatory and immunosuppressive effects in the human body. Several different pathways are affected by these medications. Glucocorticoids reduce macrophage phagocytosis, IL-2 secretion, and number of monocytes. They also inhibit prostaglandin and leukotriene synthesis and the release of collagenase and lysosomal enzymes.[14] Glucocorticoids can be administered through oral, intramuscular, intravenous, and intra-articular routes. Prednisone is given for a short period of time while the longer-term medications, such as NSAIDs and DMARDs, become effective. Typically, patients will obtain greater relief from the short-term prednisone than from any other mode of treatment, such as NSAIDs.[15] The short-term therapy should be used for no longer than 6 months; if used longer, it may exacerbate the side effects typically seen with the usage of prednisone. Prednisone can interfere with glucose tolerance and therefore must be monitored very closely in patients with insulin-dependent diabetes.[16] Osteoporosis is a major concern in patients who have been on corticosteroids. The dosage of corticosteroid that is typically recommended is less than 10 mg/day; also supplementation with vitamin D may be helpful to maintain bone density.[5] Increase in blood pressure may also be noted, but it is unclear if this leads to significant increased risk of heart disease or stroke.[16]

Pulse therapy using methylprednisolone has been used in the treatment of acute flares. It takes about 6 to 8 weeks to respond to this therapy. So, this therapy is often used as a last line of treatment for patients with RA.[17]

Intra-articular therapy is also an important method of delivering medication to RA sites. This therapy is not disease modifying; however, it does provide analgesic care. Several medications can be used to help treat RA, including hydrocortisone succinate, and triamcinolone hexacetonide. After the injection, the patient is recommended to rest for a period of 24 hours. Chakravarty and colleagues[14] showed in a randomized controlled study that patients who rested for 24 hours after their injection had much greater pain relief 12 weeks postinjection than patients who did not. Injections come with their own set of complications, and care must be taken when using intra-articular therapy. Tendon rupture and osteonecrosis can be potential side effects from this treatment modality.

When using glucocorticoids in patients with RA, it is important to pay attention to how long and how often patients are given their pharmacotherapy. Jain and Lipsky[18] suggest from many studies that this type of therapy should be used as a temporary therapy until a more long-term therapy can become effective.

As research continues on the treatment methods for RA, new therapies are being developed and tested. Several newer advances that have been thought of, but not yet tested or approved, include the use of statin medications for their antiinflammatory effects and the use of stem cell therapy.[19] Until more research is done, practitioners should continue using the available methods for treating RA. Foot and ankle specialists and rheumatologists should work hand in hand to manage patients with RA.

NONPHARMACOLOGIC THERAPY
Joint Protective Modalities

The initial chief complaint of a patient with RA is pain. This pain causes an unstable gait and enhances other preexisting foot abnormalities in these patients. Their gait velocity is decreased, causing lesser time in single limb stance.[20] The heel also tends to be everted with prolonged subtalar joint pronation through midstance while typically having a painful hallux valgus deformity. Body weight is transferred posteriorly, causing a late heel rise and lesser time in single limb stance. Patients are also reluctant in the push-off phase because of painful metatarsal head subluxation and hammer-toe abnormalities. Heel contact is often painful because of retrocalcaneal bursitis, super-ficial calcaneal bursitis, and/or heel spurs.[20] These conditions are all indications for joint protective measures, which include custom-made foot orthoses, splints, paddings, and custom-made extra-depth shoe gear, all of which help to minimize pressure, reduce shock and sheer forces, support or improve deformities, and control or decrease pain.[21]

Kavlak and colleagues[20] demonstrated in a 3-month-study that custom foot orthoses and custom shoe gear affected pain, gait, and physiologic cost index (energy expenditure), with P-value results less than 0.05 regarding all parameters, such as decrease in pain, increase in step length and stride length, and reduction in energy expenditure. Data analysis by "Student t test for repeated measurements was used and p value was set up as 0.05 for statistical analysis of data with the SPSS (Statistical Package for Social Sciences) for Windows Release 6.0 statistical packet program."[20] Physiologic cost index calculates the energy used by a patient during ambulation, which is essential for evaluating the benefits of custom foot orthoses and custom shoe gear on gait efficiency.[20]

A 12-week randomized control study, discussed in a systematic review by Farrow and colleagues,[22] demonstrated higher degrees of pain relief from metatarsalgia for patients wearing extra-depth shoegear with semirigid inserts than for those wearing the shoes alone or with soft inserts.

A 6-week case study by Shrader and Siegel[23] was conducted on a 55-year-old women with a 10-year history of RA who complained of ongoing painful functional hallux limitus (FHL) bilaterally with greater left toe pain. The patient's FHL pain progressively worsened and interfered with ADLs, and she soon began 4 sessions of physical therapy (PT). During each individual session, the patient was fitted for semi-rigid orthoses, custom shoe gear, modifications to shoe gear, and patient education. After PT and no change in rheumatoid medications, her FHL pain was completely resolved as a result of using custom orthoses and custom shoe gear. The patient was able to walk for 4 hours without pain after treatment, whereas previously she could walk only for 30 minutes without pain. Left hallux peak plantar pressures were reduced from 43 to 18 N/cm^2.

Other protective measures for joints are discussed in more detail later in the article for resultant soft tissue disorders of RA, including rheumatoid nodules, tarsal tunnel syndrome, plantar fasciitis, retrocalcaneal bursitis, tenosynovitis, complete tendon rupture, and posterior tibial tendon dysfunction.

Rheumatoid nodules can be found overlying any bony protuberance and the Achilles tendon and plantar fat pad site. These rheumatoid nodules rub against the shoe gear, resulting in friction and causing skin irritation. Treatment should include orthoses and soft donut-shaped padding to off-load the pressure of the nodule.[19]

Hyperkeratotic tissue or hard callus is a common feature overlying hammer toes, rheumatoid nodules, and subluxed metatarsal heads, causing significant pain. Care of these simple yet painful dermatologic lesions includes debridement followed by use of adhesive felt pad, tube foam, and/or silipos tubing. To avoid progressive forma-tion of calluses, patients' shoe gear should accommodate the foot deformities with an extra-depth toe box, a low soft heel, a firm heel counter, and a lace-up style upper with plastizote inserts.[1] A plastizote insert is made up of closed-cell polyethylene foam, which can be molded to the foot by heating the insert in a microwave for about 10 to 20 seconds. These inserts relieve pressure in the arthritic joints and aid in the prevention of ulcerations in patients with RA and diabetes.[24] However, these inserts should be replaced every few months because they bottom out while accommodating to the pressures associated with forefoot deformities.[25]

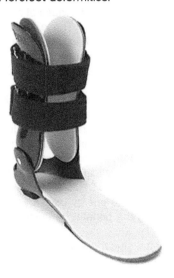

Pictured above are plastizote inserts placed on an ankle foot orthosis (AFO) device.

Superficial calcaneal bursitis can be treated with an elevated or no-heel counter within the modified shoe gear along with a silicone pad to cover the irritated skin overlying the protuberant bursa. In retrocalcaneal bursitis, a heel lift can be used in the patient's shoes.[4]

A patient with RA typically acquires a planovalgus deformity and is subjected to tibial nerve traction or entrapment and can subsequently develop tarsal tunnel syndrome. Modified orthoses with medial rearfoot posting to counteract the hindfoot valgus is indicated for treatment and immobilization, to decrease pressure off the soft tissues, resulting in decreased inflammation.[4]

Plantar fasciitis should be treated with gastroc-soleus and plantar fascia stretching, icing, orthoses modified with a heel cup, night splints, and (in more severe cases) extracorporeal shock wave therapy and/or cast immobilization.[4]

Tenosynovitis is very common in patients with RA. In mild to moderate cases, treatment should consist of orthotics and PT. If inflammation does not resolve and the tendon sheath thickens or completely ruptures, more extensive therapy should be instituted and the patient should be immobilized in a cast. For anterior tibial tendon tear, treatment should include an AFO to prevent any gait cycle abnormalities, such as the heel strike-foot slap or the swing phase-foot drag.[4] In a case at the Sisters of Charity Hospital, Buffalo, NY, a 69-year-old women presented to the clinic for a painful left foot after tripping at work. The patient had a past medical history significant for RA: degenerative joint disease, lumbar spinal stenosis, glaucoma, and macular degeneration. She had earlier consulted an orthopedic surgeon who treated her conservatively for the foot pain with fentanyl (Duragesic patch) and rofecoxib (Vioxx) and Dynastep (Brown Shoe Co, Clayton, MO, USA) insoles for metatarsalgia. Patient's symptoms never improved. This patient was then referred to a neurologist who treated her with gabapentin (Neurontin) for idiopathic neuropathy. In 2009, the patient fell and had reported instability upon ambulation. Physical examination revealed that dorsalis pedis and posterior tibial pulses were palpable. Muscle strength of 3/5 for dorsiflexors of the left leg was observed. All other muscle groups measured 5/5. Deep tendon reflex at the Achilles tendon revealed a strength of 2/4. Negative Hohman sign observed was bilateral. There was a palpable mass at the dorsal medial aspect of the left foot with decreased dorsiflexion. Plain-film radiographs were consistent with arthritic changes in the left foot. The patient was sent for magnetic resonance imaging (MRI) of the left foot. The image results as seen in **Fig. 1** show a complete rupture of the tibialis anterior tendon retracted at the level of the tibial plafond. Also seen on the MRI were tendinopathy and longitudinal split tearing of the peroneus brevis tendon and minimal tearing of the Achilles tendon. Surgical and nonsurgical options were discussed with the patient, and it was determined to continue the nonsurgical options, including rest, icing, and elevation. The patient was placed in a cam walker (Alimed Inc, Dedham, MA, USA) until an AFO could be made (**Fig. 2**).

According to the posterior tibial tendon dysfunction (PTTD) classification system developed by Johnson and Strom, stages 1 to 4 for PTTD[26] indicate the tendon's severity of dysfunction and treatment options. In the initial stage, there is no deformity, and over-the-counter orthotics are sufficient treatment. Earlier stages include a minor deformity of flexible pes planovalgus, and treatment consists of custom-made semi-rigid arch supports, such as Spenco (Spenco Medical Corp, Waco, TX, USA), which is modified with rearfoot medial posting and medial longitudinal arch support to combat the pronator forces along with an ankle brace (elastic, stirrup, or lace-up). Spenco is made up of a nylon (plastic) arch support, covered in green neoprene cushioned material measuring 9.58 mm in depth. These arch supports correct both medial and lateral arches in patients who have very flat feet and are more comfortable because of their soft top cover and flexible make compared with other more rigid arch supports. Spenco inserts are also said to reduce forefoot and rearfoot plantar pressures in comparison to barefoot walking (**Fig. 3**).[27]

In later stages with more severe deformities of the posterior tibial tendon, with or without a complete tendon rupture such as fixed planovalgus deformity and ankle

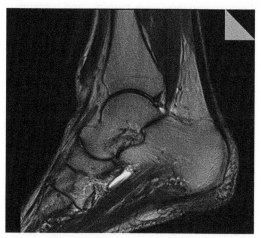

Fig. 1. A complete rupture of the tibialis anterior tendon retracted at the level of the tibial plafond.

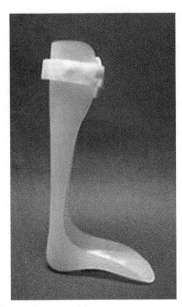

Fig. 2. A type of AFO device.

valgus deformity, treatment should include custom University of California Biomechanics Laboratory brace, solid or hinged AFO, and/or Arizona brace (**Fig. 4**).[4]

AFOs are also indicated in stabilizing the midfoot in a more rectus position by building up the lateral wall to prevent migration of the foot into an abducted position. However, patients are reluctant to wear the device because of the medial ankle irritation from the pressure point.[1]

Electrophysical Modalities

Other modalities should be considered to treat RA on a physiologic level, through electrophysical means to relieve pain and improve function. These therapies include thermotherapy, electrotherapy, low-level laser therapy, and balneotherapy.

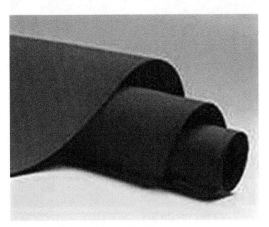

Fig. 3. Green neoprene material used to make Spenco supports.

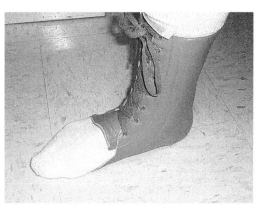

Fig. 4. Arizona brace.

Thermotherapy can be applied locally or by whole-body submersion. Therapy includes a cold or hot source or a contrast bath with cold and hot water submersions. Local application of a cold (ice packs, ice chips, ice massage, cryowraps, cold air, or vapocoolant sprays) or a hot (superficial heat, such as hot packs, paraffin or wax baths, and infrared, and deep heat, such as electromagnetic wave forms and ultrasound)[21] source can be used to provide short-term pain relief and to decrease joint stiffness, whereas paraffin wax baths provide more long-term results according to the British Society of Rheumatology (BSR) and British Health Professionals in Rheumatology (BHPR).[21] However, Ayling and Marks evaluated the efficacy of paraffin wax baths in 4 randomized control trials (RCTs) (303 participants), with little evidence to support its use in treatment and with no concrete methods on optimal application. The results suggested that paraffin wax could be temporarily useful or not useful at all, and it should be avoided in patients with active RA. Nonetheless, many reviews for thermotherapy have suggested that its use in conjunction with other therapies, that is, pharmacologic therapy and foot orthoses, can be beneficial.[3] The Ottawa Panel reviewed 2 RCTs (76 participants) on the effects of thermotherapy, especially the use of paraffin wax as an adjunct to exercise, and showed high-quality evidence relating to pain and stiffness relief with increased joint range of motion (ROM).[3] The high-level evidence equates to "one or more updated, high-quality systematic reviews that are based on at least 2 high-quality primary studies with consistent results."[3]

Therapeutic ultrasound delivers high-frequency mechanical vibrations in either a continuous fashion to relieve pain by its thermal effects or by pulsed sequence to decrease inflammation. The heating effects of continuous ultrasound can also reduce muscle spasms and stimulate blood flow to help decrease inflammatory toxins. A flexibility program can also be instilled earlier on in the disease process because ultrasound can penetrate deeper tissues, such as collagen, to increase its elasticity.[28] Ottawa Panel reviewed the use of therapeutic ultrasound in 1 RCT (50 participants) that had a mean quality Jadad score of 3.0 (Jadad scale 0–5) and showed high-quality evidence that ultrasound significantly decreases painful joints and increases function.[3]

Using contrast baths is another thermal modality to decrease inflammation, swelling, pain, and joint stiffness. A systematic review was done on the effectiveness of contrast baths, where volunteers' affected joints were submersed into hot water and then into cold water, with variation in temperature, time, and duration to test the more effective reaction time.[29] The best bathing time was 6 minutes in hot water followed by 4 minutes in cold water, but some preferred a 4:1 ratio of hot water to cold water submersion for the best physiologic effect on blood flow. The preferred temperatures were 106°F to 113°F for hot water submersion and 47°F to 60°F for cold water submersion. Study results indicated that there was no physiologic effect on intramuscular temperature and the lymphatic system, whereby there was no change in lymphatic edema. However, with contrast bathing, there was an increase in skin temperature and superficial blood flow down to the subcutaneous level. Contrast bathing may be contraindicated in patients having Raynaud phenomenon.[25]

Cold and hot thermotherapies, including cryotherapy, infrared sauna, and thermal baths, can also be used for whole-body treatment.[21]

Electrotherapy Modalities

Electrotherapy is used to control pain and to increase muscle strength and function. One form of electrotherapy often used is the transcutaneous electrical nerve stimulation (TENS), in which there are 3 different ways of administering electric current: conventional TENS (C-TENS), acupuncture-like TENS (AL-TENS), and burst TENS.[30] Electrical current is transmitted through electrodes to a specific muscle of interest to stimulate motor units.[3,21] The C-TENS transmits an electric current of high frequency with a low intensity, allowing for immediate pain relief, but is effective only when the TENS unit is still turned on. The AL-TENS uses a current of low frequency with a high intensity, which has been found to be painful or uncomfortable for patients. The burst TENS uses high frequency burst impulses at a low intensity.[30] Burst TENS is believed to be beneficial in providing pain relief by stimulating pain-carrying fibers and allowing a comfortable treatment process because of the high internal frequency.[31]

Even though there are studies on the use of TENS for the treatment of only hand problems in patients with RA, it should be another modality to be considered within the foot and ankle specialist community also. The BSR and the BHPR agree that the use of TENS is beneficial for reducing pain in the patient with RA, but this concept lacks standardization.[21] Another study consisting of 3 RCTs (78 participants) evaluated by Brosseau and colleagues[30] on the use of TENS unit for treatment of RA in the hands also found good evidence, with a mean quality Jadad score of 2.3. Brosseau and colleagues state that "there are conflicting effects on pain outcomes in patients with RA. AL-TENS is beneficial for reducing pain intensity and improving muscle power scores over placebo, while conversely, C-TENS resulted in no clinical benefit on pain intensity compared with placebo. However, C-TENS resulted in a clinical benefit on patient assessment of change in disease over AL-TENS." Therefore, patients believed that the C-TENS helped decrease their intensity of pain best.

Low-level laser therapy is another modality to relieve pain and to improve function in patients with RA. The laser emits a single wavelength of pure light, which causes a photochemical reaction within the cell.[3,21] A study consisting of 5 RCTs (204 participants), with a Jadad mean quality score of 4.0 and reviewed by the Ottawa panel, noted that 3 of the RCTs revealed significant improvements in pain and 2 RCTs found moderate quality of increased ROM and flexibility.[3] Moderate level of evidence is based on "one high-quality primary study or with two primary studies of moderate quality with consistent results."[3] No side effects or safety precautions were addressed.

After summarizing the current literature, it was found that there have been very few systematic reviews done on the effectiveness of these electrophysical therapeutic treatments and that most of these studies are not geared toward RA. So, further research should be considered.

Exercise and Physical Activity

All the above-mentioned modalities can facilitate therapeutic benefits in patients with RA. In addition, implementation of exercises and physical activities can be a beneficial adjunct to their current pharmaceutical treatments, which can help increase muscle strength, ROM, and endurance. Exercising, for the management of RA is agreed upon by the European League against Rheumatism, the BSR and the BHPR.[21] Exercise helps maintain physical fitness by having the patient participate in repetitive, structured workouts. However, dynamic exercise is best suited for patients with RA because it permits for tolerable intensity, duration, and frequency to increase muscle strength and fitness potential, without exacerbating the arthritic joints and causing increase in pain.[21] The BSR and the BHPR recommend the following exercises for patients with RA to manage their debilitating symptoms: (1) ROM exercises to improve joint mobility and decrease joint stiffness, (2) resistance-based workouts to increase muscle strength, and (3) aerobic activity to increase overall fitness.[2] An evidence-based review conducted by Oldfield and Felson[2] showed that aerobic activity of moderate intensity done 3 times a week and strengthening workouts of increased intensity done 2 to 3 times a week, all from 30 to 60 minutes, are beneficial for patients with RA.

The BSR and the BHPR also have evidence showing that hydrotherapy, such as pool exercise, not only decreases pain and improves function but also improves health-related quality of life. Along with exercise or a community-based PT program, integrating education on RA to patients will instill the importance of exercise to maintain pain-free motion and muscle strength. Physical therapists found that when patients had an increased awareness and knowledge of RA, they showed self-improvement and a decrease in morning stiffness.[21] Unfortunately, there is no current evidence that exercise can affect disease regression or progression. Follow-ups from 12 to 24 weeks to 1 year have shown that land-based aerobic exercises had no effect in the improvement or worsening of RA.[2]

Patients with RA should be managed not only by their rheumatologist but also by an established team of care workers, such as foot and ankle specialists, orthopedic surgeons, physical therapists, occupational therapists, nurse specialists, dieticians, and social workers. A review consisting of 15 controlled clinical trials (9 were RCTs) concluded that care of inpatients by a multidisciplinary team of workers had the same level of effectiveness as that of day-patient care and surpassed the effectiveness of outpatient care. Nonetheless, 2 RCTs noted that inpatient care is more expensive than day-patient care.[21]

Occupational and physical therapists, according to the BSR and the BHPR, are indicated to improve self-management strategies in patients with RA who experience trouble at work because of their arthritis.[21] As a result of the progressive nature of RA, patients have an early decrease in their ADLs, and most are unable to hold a job within 2 years of diagnosis; so referral to an occupational therapist is recommended. Therapists can institute training techniques, such as pacing (energy conservation), posture, training of motor function, and instruction on joint-protective assisted devices (splints, orthoses), to help patients manage their debilitating disease and function better at work.[3,21] To increase the patient's independence during ambulation, it is important to refer to PT for gait training. Further, depending on the upper body involvement in the RA, patients would be given modified handicap-aiding equipments, such as platform crutches or canes with special handgrips. Therapists can also assist in stretching exercises with passive or active manipulation of the ankle joint for a con-tracted Achilles tendon and for the metatarsal phalangeal and interphalangeal joints for contracted digits to maintain motion. Muscle strengthening and conditioning also helps to maintain function in early RA.[25]

COMPLIMENTARY AND ALTERNATIVE MEDICINE THERAPY

Because of the persistent and progressive nature of RA, patients are more likely to seek out other treatments in hopes that it will benefit their current regimen of drug therapy and other conservative measures taken during the course of their disease. This is called CAM therapy, where complimentary medicine is used in conjunction with current medicine, and alternative medicine replaces current or conventional medicine.[3] Patients tend to seek out herbs and vitamins and alter their diet. They also seek homeopathy treatments (such as passive hydrotherapy, also known as bal-neotherapy), movement therapies (such as tai chi), and other eastern medicines (such as acupuncture).

Diet control is not a usual prerequisite in the treatment of RA. The BSR and the BHPR state that patients with RA have an increased risk of cardiovascular disease (CVD).[21] Clinical practice guidelines for RA also state that patients with RA have an increased risk of CVD and that patients with comorbidities such as diabetes, obesity, and osteoporosis should be treated with proper nutrition. Therapies such as elimina-tion diets in early RA should be discouraged.[21] However, a review of 2 RCTs, consis-tent with moderate quality, reported that fasting followed by a vegetarian diet for 3 months resulted in decreased pain. There was no mention of any negative effect on patients' health due to preliminary fasting.[3] Other studies have indicated that patients have an increased risk of RA if intake of fruits and vegetables and antioxidants, such as vitamin C and B-cryptoxanthin, are significantly low.[21] It is also indicated that patients with RA tend to have a lower serum carotenoid level, which is found in fruits and vege-tables, and this low level of serum antioxidants could be a risk factor for CVD.[21]

Fish oil supplemented in the diet is said to decrease pain and morning stiffness. The efficacy of fish oil has been tested at higher doses, whereby 1 to 7 g/d of fish oil is indi-cated for 3 months for the proper intake of this supplement. A meta-analysis RCT was conducted, which noted that fish oil was made up of long-chain omega (n)-3 polyun-saturated fatty acids and eicosapentaenoic acid plus docosahexaenoic acid, all of which have analgesic properties, particularly the n-3 fatty acids that provide modest decrease in inflammatory joint pain.[21] Based on past reviewed trials, patients are indi-cated to take 3.5 g of n-3 fatty acids per day, which is up to 4 to 6 capsules.[21]

Because RA patients are at a higher risk for osteoporosis, they are recommended to have an adequate intake of calcium and vitamin D of 700 to 1000 mg/d as preventative medicine.[21]

Herbal therapy such as intake of gamma-linolenic acid (GLA) was reviewed in 3 RCTs of moderate quality, which concluded that this herb reduces pain and improves patient global assessment.[3] "Three studies showing fewer clinical responses provided a relatively low daily dosage of GLA (between 525 and 540 mg) for a duration of only 6 to 12 weeks. By comparison, 3 studies that used doses between 1.4 and 2.8 g GLA for a duration of 24 weeks reported greater improvements in symptoms of arthritis. In 1 trial people who went on with GLA for a second 6 months continued to show improve-ment. Five of the GLA studies reported adverse reactions and many of these were related to digestive upset."[32]

Although balneotherapy, also known as spa therapy or passive hydrotherapy, has positive findings, there is no sufficient evidence proving that this therapy reduces pain and increases function. This is because of its poor methodologic quality, which lacks thorough statistical analysis and therefore has no positive effects for benefiting the patient.[3,21] Balneotherapy consists of mudpacks, sulfur baths, Dead Sea salt baths, and/or bathing in water with minerals.[3]

It is already known that patients with RA have a decrease in muscle strength and joint ROM, which affects their way of ambulating and is worsened by the ongoing inflammatory destruction of their joints. That is why many patients try the traditional Chinese martial art, tai chi. Tai chi focuses on balance and good posture with slow movements while performing deep breathing in a bent-knee squat position. Because the exercise is weight-bearing, it could stimulate bony growth. According to a synthesized research, Han and colleagues[33] noted that there was increased lower-extremity joint ROM, especially in the ankle joint. The increased flexibility of the joints could be attributed to the exercise strengthening the surrounding connective tissue.

Another traditional Chinese homeopathic treatment is the use of acupuncture for medical conditions. Acupuncture can help reduce pain and stress and equalize internal energy. Needles are placed within the skin at certain points, where they are manipulated either by fingers or by a small electrical current (known as electroacupuncture). Casimiro and colleagues[34] discussed symptomatic knee pain in patients with RA who had a minimal amount of pain reduction 4 months after acupuncture.

RA is a multisystem disease presenting itself 90% of the time in the foot and ankle, and foot and ankle specialists are the first to diagnose this condition and make appropriate referrals or begin medical treatment.[35] The early conservative use of pharmacologic and nonpharmacologic therapy instilled within the treatment regimen of the patient with RA will help provide pain relief, improve mobility, and increase ADLs. Some of the compiled literature mentioned earlier had weak evidence because of limitations within its study. This indicates that further research is required to provide definitive conclusions on the use of the above conservative treatments. Other studies had sufficient evidence to provide information to best treat patients with RA in a timely manner with appropriate palliative treatment, such as pharmacologic therapy and custom-made foot orthoses, braces, and shoe modifications. Comanagement with other medical physicians on the proper treatment of the RA patient can help control the disease process and avoid surgical intervention.

REFERENCES

1. Jaakkola J, Mann R. A review of rheumatoid arthritis affecting the foot and ankle. Foot Ankle Int 2004;25(12):866–74.
2. Oldfield V, Felson DT. Exercise therapy and orthotic devices in rheumatoid arthritis: evidence-based review. Curr Opin Rheumatol 2008;20:353–9.
3. Christie A, Jamtvedt G, Thuve Dahm K, et al. Effectiveness of nonpharmacological and nonsurgical interventions for patient with rheumatoid arthritis: an overview of systemic reviews. Phys Ther 2007;87:12.
4. Aronow M, Hakim-Zargar M. Management of hindfoot disease in rheumatoid arthritis. Foot Ankle Clin 2007;12:455–74.
5. Drugs for rheumatoid arthritis. Treat Guidel Med Lett 2009;7(81):37–46.
6. Simon L. The COX 2 selective inhibitors: what the newspapers have not told you. Bull NYU Hosp Jt Dis 2007;65(3):229.
7. McKellar G, Madhok R, Singh G. The problem with NSAIDs: what data to believe. Curr pain headache rep 2007;11:423–7.

8. Shi S, Klotz U. Clinical use and pharmacological properties of selective COX-2 inhibitors. Eur J Clin Pharmacol 2008;62:233–52.

9. Saag KG, Teng GG, Patkar NM, et al. American college of rheumatology recommendations for the use of nonbiologic and biologic disease-modifying antirheumatic drugs in rheumatoid arthritis. Arthritis Rheum 2008;59:762.

10. Bingham C, Miner M. Treatment, management, and monitoring of established rheumatoid arthritis. J Fam Pract 2007;56:S1–7.

11. Cronstein BN. Molecular therapeutics: methotrexate and its mechanism of action. Arthritis Rheum 1951;1996:39.

12. Plushner S. Tocilizumab: an interleukin-6 receptor inhibitor for the treatment of rheumatoid arthritis. Ann Pharmacother 2008;42:1660–8.

13. Buttgereit F, Straub RH, Wehling M, et al. Glucocorticoids in the treatment of rheumatic disease: an update on the mechanisms of action. Arthritis Rheum 2004;50:3408.

14. Chakravarty K, Pharoah PDP, Scott DGI. A randomized controlled study of post-injection rest following intra-articular steroid therapy for knee synovitis. Br J Rheumatol 1994;33:464–8.

15. Gotzsche PC, Johansen HK. Meta-analysis of short-term low dose prednisolone versus placebo and non-sterodial anti-inflammatory drugs in rheumatoid arthritis. BMJ 1998;316:811.

16. Cohen MD, Conn DL. Benefits of low-dose corticosteroids in rheumatoid arthritis. Bull Rheum Dis 1997;46(4):4–7.

17. Smith MD, Ahern MJ, Roberts-Thompson PJ. Pulse methylprednisone therapy in rheumatoid arthritis: unproved therapy, unjustified therapy, or effective adjunctive treatment. Ann Rheum Dis 1990;49:265.

18. Jain R, Lipsky PE. Treatment of rheumatoid arthritis. Med Clin North Am 1997;81:57.

19. Arnaud C, Mach F. Potential anti-inflammatory and immunomodulatory effects of statins in rheumatological therapy. Arthritis Rheum 2006;54:390.

20. Kavlak Y, Uygur F, Korkmaz C, et al. Outcome of orthoses intervention in rheumatoid foot. Foot Ankle Int 2003;23(6):494–9.

21. Vlieland T, Pattison D. Non-drug therapies in early rheumatoid arthritis. Best Pract Res Clin Rheumatol 2009;23:103–16.

22. Farrow S, Kingsley G, Scott D. Interventions for foot disease in rheumatoid arthritis: a systemic review. Arthritis Rheum 2005;53(4):595–602.

23. Shrader J, Siegel K. Nonoperative management of functional hallux limitus in a patient with rheumatoid arthritis. Phys Ther 2003;83(9):831–43.

24. Lord M, Hosein R. Pressure redistribution by molded inserts in diabetic footwear: a pilot study. J Rehabil R D 1994;31(3):214–21.

25. Coughlin MJ, Mann RA, Saltzman C. Arthritic conditions of the foot. In: Coughlin MJ, Mann RA, Saltzman C, editors. Surgery of the Foot and Ankle, vol. 1. 8th edition. Philadelphia: Mosby Elsevier; 2007. p. 816–17, Chapter 16.

26. Kohls-Gatzoulis J, Angel J, Singh D, et al. Tibialis posterior dysfunction: a common and treatable cause of adult acquired flatfoot. BMJ 2004;329:1328–33.

27. McPoil TG, Cornwall MW. Effect of insole material on force and plantar pressures during walking. J Am Podiatr Med Assoc 1992;82(8):412–6.

28. Casimiro L, Brosseau L, Robinson V, et al. Therapeutic ultrasound for the treatment of rheumatoid arthritis. Cochrane Database Syst Rev 2002;(3):CD003787.

29. Stanton D, Lazaro R, MacDermid J. A systematic review of the effectiveness of contrasts baths. J Hand Ther 2009;22:57–70.

30. Brosseau L, Yonge KA, Welch V, et al. Transcutaneous electrical nerve stimulation (TENS) for the treatment of rheumatoid arthritis in the hand. Cochrane Database Syst Rev 2009;3:1–20.

31. Imboden J, Hellmann D, Stone J. Transcutaneous electrical nerve stimulation. Current Rheumatology Diagnosis & Treatment 2006;2:454.

32. Little CV, Parsons T. Herbal therapy for treating rheumatoid arthritis. Cochrane Database Syst Rev 2000;(4):CD002948.

33. Han A, Judd MG, Robinson VA, et al. Tai chi for treating rheumatoid arthritis. Cochrane Database Syst Rev 2004;(3):CD004849.

34. Casimiro L, Barnsley L, Brosseau L, et al. Acupuncture and electroacupuncture for the treatment of rheumatoid arthritis. Cochrane Database Syst Rev 2005;(4): CD003788.

35. Costa M, Rizak T, Zimmermann B. Rheumatologic conditions of the foot. J Am Podiatr Med Assoc 2004;94:177–86.

Medical Imaging and Radiographic Analysis of the Rheumatoid Patient

Adam Hicks, DPM[a], Heiko Adams, DPM[a,b,*],
Jeffrey Szczepanski, DPM[c]

KEYWORDS

• Rheumatoid arthritis • Imaging • Radiographic analysis • Foot

Historically, rheumatoid arthritis (RA) has been diagnosed using the classification system developed by the American College of Rheumatology, wherein at least 4 out of 7 identifiable requirements must be present for diagnosis.[1–3] Some of the criteria include symmetric arthritis, joint swelling, rheumatoid nodules, morning stiffness, positive Rh factor, and radiographic changes.[4] Radiographic assessment of RA is not only an important diagnostic criterion but also a barometer for disease progression. Advanced arthritic change is a clear indicator of disease progression, requiring changes in the current treatment regimen. Radiographic classifications are thus important in the diagnosis and staging of the disease progression.

Many researchers have attempted to decrease the interobserver versus intraobserver variability associated with diagnosing and monitoring RA. In 1949, Steinbrocker and colleagues[5] used 4 stages of a single isolated joint to describe radiographic changes. This system identified osteoporosis, erosions, bone and cartilage destruction, and finally ankylosis as the key characteristics for grading. This staging system lacked a key fundamental aspect of RA, because it assessed only one joint for radiographic diagnosis.

In 1971, Sharp and colleagues[6] scored the progression of arthritic changes in an attempt to evaluate the effect of therapy on those affected. Sharp and colleagues[6] used a retrospective study to identify 10 key features of RA in the hands and wrist: periosteal reaction, cortical thinning, osteoporosis, sclerosis, osteophyte formation, defects, cystic changes, surface erosions, joint-space narrowing, and ankylosis.

[a] Jewish Hospital and St Mary's Healthcare Podiatric Residency Program, Louisville, KY, USA
[b] Private Practice, Shelbyville, KY, USA
[c] Private Practice, Traverse City, MI, USA
* Corresponding author. Jewish Hospital and St Mary's Healthcare Podiatric Residency Program, Louisville, KY.
E-mail address: footdoc@insightbb.com

Clin Podiatr Med Surg 27 (2010) 209–218
doi:10.1016/j.cpm.2009.12.009   **podiatric.theclinics.com**
0891-8422/10/$ – see front matter © 2010 Elsevier Inc. All rights reserved.

The investigators ruled out 8 of the 10 diagnostic factors and concluded that 2 scores were best used to evaluate progression: one being defects and destruction and the other being joint-space narrowing. It was also acknowledged that joint swelling was a distinctive characteristic, and was hence added to the scoring system at a later date. The study also showed a direct correlation between increased Rh factor titers and noted radiographic changes.

In 1977, Larsen and colleagues[7] evaluated the radiographic assessment of RA that had been carried out previously by the aforementioned investigators as well as the staging system that he had published previously. The present study highlighted the interobserver discrepancies that make radiographic evaluation of RA so difficult. The Larsen grading system incorporated a grade 0, which described normal conditions, with no abnormalities related to arthritis. Grade I had slight abnormality with one or more lesions noted, including periarticular-tissue swelling, periarticular osteoporosis, and slight joint-space narrowing. Progressive grades II, III, and IV transitioned from a definite abnormality to severe deformity. Grade V was described as a mutilating deformity. Anatomically, this study evaluated multiple joints, including proximal and distal interphalangeal joints of the hand, metacarpo- and metatarsophalangeal joints, the wrist, the elbow, the shoulder, the hip, the ankle, the subtalar joint, and the hallux interphalangeal joint.

Rau and colleagues[8] attempted to improve the reliability and to define the minimal detectable change in RA in a better manner. Rau brought Sharp and Larsen together to form a panel that reviewed previous scoring methods. The new staging method decided on attributes from previous studies carried out by both Larsen and Sharp. The new method, instead of scoring the number or size of joint erosions, measured the total joint-surface destruction. Joint destruction is defined by the length of the clear visible interruption of the cortical plate in relation to the total joint surface. Based on the percentage of joint-surface destruction the grading system is as follows: Grade 1, less then 20%; Grade 2, 21% to 40%; Grade 3, 41% to 60%; Grade 4, 61% to 80%; Grade 5, greater than 80%. A total of 38 joints including 10 proximal interphalangeal joints, 10 metacarpophalangeal joints, 4 sites in the wrist, metatarsophalangeal joints 2 to 5, and bilateral hallux interphalangeal joints were used for evaluation. The hypothesis of this study was to create a more reliable grading method, which was illustrated by measuring the minimal detectable changes between radiographs and between multiple readers. The results surpassed both Sharp's and Larsen's previous attempts.

CONVENTIONAL RADIOGRAPHY

Conventional radiography (CR) has long been considered the gold standard for the diagnosis and prognosis of RA. The relative ease with which a radiograph can be obtained versus the time and effort that is required to perform magnetic resonance imaging (MRI), allows CR to continue its relevance. In 2008, Ostergaard and colleagues[9] described the advantages and disadvantages of CR. These investigators stated that the advantages included "low cost, high availability, possibility of standardization, blinded-centralized reading, reasonable reproducibility, and existence of validated assessment methods"; whereas the disadvantages included "projectional superimposition caused by the 2-dimensional representation of 3-dimensional pathology, use of ionizing radiation, relative insensitivity to early bone damage, and total insufficiency for assessment of soft-tissue changes including synovitis."[9] Scoring criteria that has been previously mentioned will still be used as research guidelines against which all other future studies will be compared. Because the treatment paradigm for RA is early diagnosis and intervention, the value of radiography has been significantly decreased for this capacity. Standard radiography is still considered the gold standard by most podiatric surgeons to guide surgical care for these patients.

Fig. 1A, B show pre- and postoperative radiographs of surgical forefoot reconstruction. Standard anteroposterior weight-bearing images are included. In most podiatric practices, standard radiology is used to assess the disease involvement, not the disease progression. Rheumatologists mainly use standard radiographs of the hands and feet to monitor disease progression and response to treatment. Most podiatric physicians use radiographs in surgical planning.

MRI

Current treatment protocols have elucidated the need for early detection of arthritic changes using MRI. MRI has become a clear predictor of future erosive changes seen on radiographs. In a 2-year randomized, double-blinded, clinical study of patients with early RA, Hetland and colleagues[10] showed that MRI edema scores were significantly associated with radiographic progression after 2 years. This study assessed prognostic factors, including MRI, CR, and immunologic, environmental, genetic, and disease-activity markers. Of all the factors examined, bone marrow edema identified by MRI was the highest prognostic predictor of future radiographic erosions (**Figs. 2** and **3**).

In a prospective 1-year follow-up study by Haavardsholm and colleagues,[11] serial MRI images of the wrist were compared with conventional radiographs. All of the patients were being pharmacologically treated with either disease-modifying antirheumatic drugs (DMARDs) or antitumor necrosis factor, with most patients also being administered corticosteroids. The Rheumatoid Arthritis Magnetic Resonance Imaging System (RAMRIS) scoring method was used to score the joints over a 1-year period. Again, the best predictor of progressive joint destruction and benefits of DMARDs was bone marrow edema. The investigators concluded that a RAMRIS bone marrow edema score greater than 2 increased the risk of CR progression threefold.

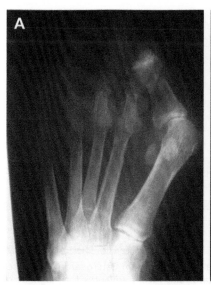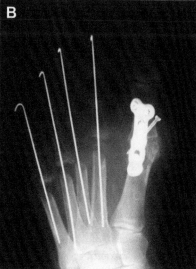

Fig. 1. Standard plain film anteroposterior (*A*) preoperative and (*B*) postoperative radiographs. (*From* private collection, Jeffrey Szczepanski, DPM, FACFAS; with permission.)

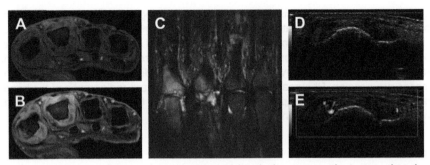

Fig. 2. A comparison of (*A, B, C*) MR images and (*D, E*) ultrasonography images that show synovitis in the metacarpal joints. (*From* Ostergaard M, Pedersen S, Dohn U. Imaging in rheumatoid arthritis—status and recent advances for magnetic resonance imaging, ultrasonography, computed tomography, and conventional radiography. Best Pract Res Clin Rheumatol 2008;22(6):1019–44; with permission.)

Determination of treatment effectiveness is the key to long-term outcomes in patients with RA. Clinical findings and serologic studies give some indication of treatment results, but imaging studies determine the actual disease state and progression. Therefore, the OMERACT-RAMRIS scoring system has been devised so that disease progression as well as interobserver coordination can be monitored and made more effective. The OMERACT-RAMRIS scoring system has been developed by the Committee on Outcome Measures in Rheumatoid Arthritis Clinical Trials (OMERACT), which has defined various MRI findings and has provided a scoring system that has been well accepted throughout the medical community. The group also delivered a reference atlas for scoring images of synovitis, bone marrow edema, and erosion in RA in the wrist and metacarpophalangeal joints.[12]

Synovitis, bone marrow edema, and bone erosions are important pathologies associated with RA. According to Boesen and colleagues[12] important definitions of

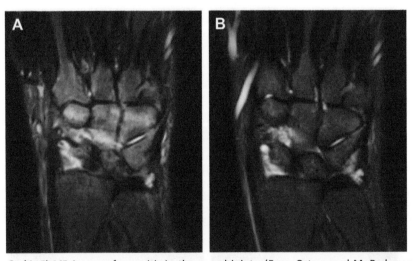

Fig. 3. (*A, B*) MR image of synovitis in the carpal joints. (*From* Ostergaard M, Pedersen S, Dohn U. Imaging in rheumatoid arthritis—status and recent advances for magnetic resonance imaging, ultrasonography, computed tomography, and conventional radiography. Best Pract Res Clin Rheumatol 2008;22(6):1019–44; with permission.)

pathologies associated with RA include synovitis, "an area in the synovial compartment that shows an above normal post-gadolinium enhancement to a thickness greater than the width of the normal synovium"; bone marrow edema, "a lesion within the trabecular bone, with ill-defined margins and signal characteristics that are consistent with increased water content"; and bone erosion, "a sharply marginated bone lesion with correct juxtaarticular localization visible in 2 planes and showing a cortical break in at least 1 plane."[12]

According to Boesen and colleagues[12] gadolinium contrast is required for better detection and scoring of synovitis pathology. It has been concluded that an overestimation of synovitis is probable without the use of contrast.[12]

Arthroscopy and synovial biopsies have validated the use of MRI for the early detection of synovitis.[13]

ULTRASONOGRAPHY

Ultrasonography (US) was first used by Cooperberg and colleagues, to describe synovitis of the knee in 1978.[14] Since that time, US has become an integral part of the rheumatologist's clinical arsenal in determining the extent of disease activity not only for synovitis but also for tenosynovitis and bone erosions.[14] In a 2007 review of the OMERACT ultrasound group it was determined that although many advances have been made to reduce the interobserver variability, there is still much research needed in long-term studies.[14] The most recent OMERACT study aimed to provide enhanced scoring methods for synovitis in the small joints of the rheumatoid arthritic hand. It was concluded that although further research is needed, an approved scoring system is possible and the need for such a system is warranted.[14]

Proponents of US as a diagnostic tool have detailed its value to the clinicians who treat rheumatic diseases. Even though MRI has become the gold standard on which all future studies could be based, US has its uses as an inexpensive 2-dimensional study that can assist in the evaluation of synovitis and joint erosions (**Figs. 4** and **5**).[15] Because CR is 2-dimensional in nature and can lag behind in tracking disease progression, US can be used to assess the effectiveness of current therapies being used. Specifically, US has been used to evaluate synovitis, which is defined as "thickened, hypoechoic, intra-articular tissue that is poorly compressible on gray-scale B-mode imaging and can show increased Doppler signals with color or power Doppler interrogation."[15] Compared with radiographic studies US has been proven to be more effective because of the real-time visualization and direct identification of bone lesions and extent of synovitis. Wakefield and colleagues[16] showed that sonography detected 127 definite erosions in 56 of 100 patients compared with 32 from radiographic identification; however, the confirmation of erosion was done via MRI. Wakefield also revealed that in early RA sonography detected 6.5-fold more erosions than did radiography.

Although not the most ideal, Ostergaard and colleagues[9] believe that this study has its advantages, such as high patient satisfaction, decreased cost, no radiation, and most importantly its capability to visualize anatomy in real time. According to Ostergaard and colleagues,[9] although US cannot penetrate bone, studies have proven that US can detect bone erosions better than CR. Although MRI has overall superiority to US, soft-tissue visualization in real time is superb, and allows easy and accurate monitoring of the synovium during DMARD administration.[9]

US imaging has the potential to visualize day-to-day progression of disease manifestations associated with RA. Because of the ease with which this imaging technique can be used, US can serve the clinician with valuable evidence on the course of the

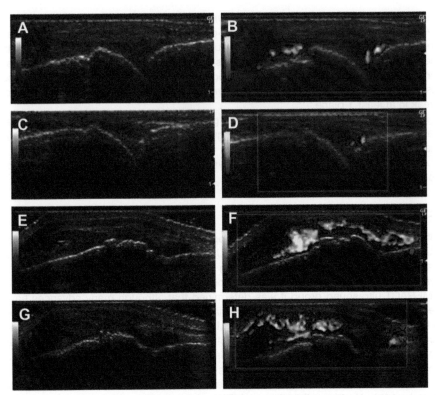

Fig. 4. A comparison of (*A, C, E, G*) standard US images and (*B, D, F, H*) color US images of synovitis. (*From* Ostergaard M, Pedersen S, Dohn U. Imaging in rheumatoid arthritis—status and recent advances for magnetic resonance imaging, ultrasonography, computed tomography, and conventional radiography. Best Pract Res Clin Rheumatol 2008;22(6):1019–44; with permission.)

disease process and benefits of current treatment. According to Ostergaard and colleagues,[9] US offers a sensitive assessment of joint damage and particularly, inflammation monitoring, and can be used by the practicing rheumatologist as part of the clinical examination.

At present, there is no specific protocol to decide which joints are to be visualized and what parameters need to be met when using US as an imaging modality. Studies have been performed, although no conclusive data are yet available.

COMPUTED TOMOGRAPHY

Computed tomography (CT) has limited use in the early detection of RA, but its clear definition of bony erosions is well documented. Although CR is still considered the gold standard, the 3-dimensional aspect of CT gives added value over CR for assessment of long-term changes to the joint surfaces (**Figs. 6** and **7**).Ostergaard and colleagues[9] believe that although CT is not readily used in the clinical setting, the ability of CT to evaluate bone erosions gives it an increased value with potential for future advances. Advantages of CT include higher sensitivity to bone erosions compared with MRI, equal radiation dose compared with CR, and the time required to obtain a CT, which is considerably shorter than the time required to obtain an

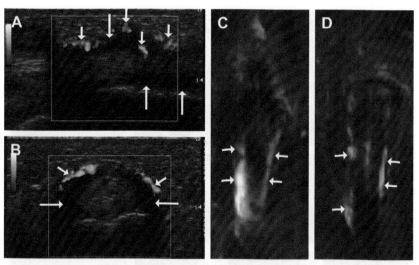

Fig. 5. A comparison of US and CR showing increased signal intensity around the joint and periosteum (*A, B, C, D*). (*From* Ostergaard M, Pedersen S, Dohn U. Imaging in rheumatoid arthritis—status and recent advances for magnetic resonance imaging, ultrasonography, computed tomography, and conventional radiography. Best Pract Res Clin Rheumatol 2008;22(6):1019–44; with permission.)

MRI.[9] Polster and colleagues[17] showed that contrast-enhanced CT can be used for the evaluation of RA and that it was comparable to MRI in the detection of synovitis, tenosynovitis, and bone erosions. In the same study it was also concluded that because of increased patient satisfaction with CT, multiple extremity scans were

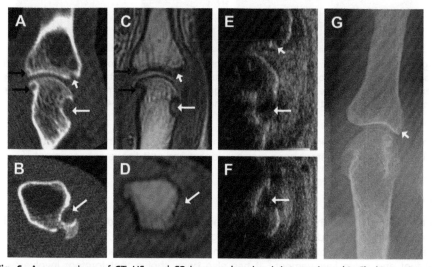

Fig. 6. A comparison of CT, US, and CR images showing joint erosions (*A–G*). (*From* Ostergaard M, Pedersen S, Dohn U. Imaging in rheumatoid arthritis—status and recent advances for magnetic resonance imaging, ultrasonography, computed tomography, and conventional radiography. Best Pract Res Clin Rheumatol 2008;22(6):1019–44; with permission.)

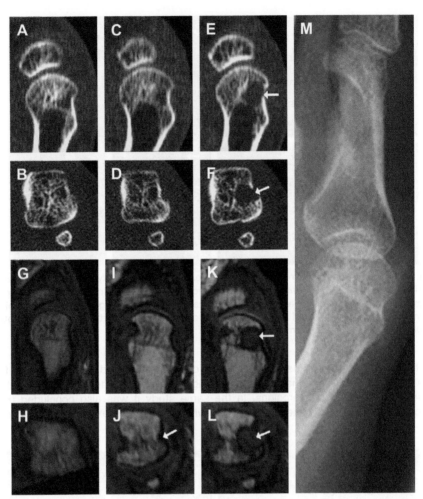

Fig. 7. A comparison of CT, US, and CR images showing joint erosions (*A–M*). (*From* Oster-gaard M, Pedersen S, Dohn U. Imaging in rheumatoid arthritis—status and recent advances for magnetic resonance imaging, ultrasonography, computed tomography, and conventional radiography. Best Pract Res Clin Rheumatol 2008;22(6):1019–44; with permission.)

possible, thus increasing the number of joints visualized.[17] The major disadvantage of CT is its inability to detect bone marrow edema and soft-tissue enhancement.[17]

SUMMARY

It has been reported that 16% to 19% of patients being treated for RA would initially present with signs and symptoms involving the foot and ankle.[2] In the same study it was shown that approximately 91% of females and 85% of males would show signs of foot and ankle involvement.[2] It has also been shown that forefoot involvement occurs much earlier in the disease process, whereas hindfoot involvement may become more apparent after the first year.[2] According to the same review, "Vidigal and colleagues reported radiographic changes in the tarsometatarsal joints in 62%

of 204 feet, only 27% of which were painful. Similarly, the subtalar joint was clinically involved in only 21% of feet, even though radiographic changes were present in 32%."[2]

As a foot and ankle physician, the diagnosis and treatment of RA takes on various forms. In many cases symptoms involving the foot and ankle can be the first signs of RA. Many times the patient will require a rheumatology consultation for systemic treatment modalities, but the overall comfort of the patient with long-standing arthritis can fall to the foot and ankle specialist. MRI has been studied extensively and the conclusion has been drawn that this imaging study is vital for the treatment of patients with RA. Although conventional radiographs are still widely used for disease progression, CT is a valid imaging modality that allows enhanced visualization of the joint erosions and thus better preoperative planning. The foot and ankle specialist has a greater anatomic appreciation for the lower extremity and its many joints. US can be used not only for disease monitoring but also for guided steroid injections, thus ensuring accurate treatment applications. According to Ostergaard and colleagues,[9] "The optimal imaging method in RA would be a sensitive and reproducible tool for diagnosis, monitoring of disease activity and damage, and prognostication."

FUTURE

The future of imaging modalities is vast for patients with RA. Because MRI is now considered the gold standard for RA, alternative methods are now being addressed. Freestone and colleagues[13] states that "cost and accessibility are still the main barriers to the widespread application of MRI in clinical practice." Hence, the study of low-field extremity MRI offers a potential solution to these barriers.[13] Cost is decreased and availability can be enhanced, but there are shortcomings because of the decreased magnetic strength and reduced clarity.[13] Studies have proven that low-field MRI has equal assessment of bony erosions, but lacks the enhanced ability of high-field MRIs for detection of synovitis.[13]

ACKNOWLEDGMENTS

We would like to thank Mikkel Østergaard for allowing permission to use diagnostic images presented in his work. We would also like to thank Diana Jackson-Adams, RT(R)ARRT for her insightful review, image selection, and help with obtaining figures.

REFERENCES

1. Arthritis foundation website. Available at: http://www.arthritis.org/disease-center.php?disease_id=31&df=diagnosed; http://www.arthritis.org/disease-center.php?disease_id=31&&df=diagnosed. Accessed December 31, 2009.
2. Jaakkola J, Mann R. A review of rheumatoid arthritis affecting the foot and ankle. FAI 2004;25(12):866–74.
3. Durez P, Malghem J, Nzeusseu A, et al. Treatment of early rheumatoid arthritis. Arthritis Rheum 2007;56(12):3919–27.
4. Arnett FC, Edworthy SM, Bloch DA, et al. The American Rheumatism Association 1987 revised criteria for the classification of rheumatoid arthritis. Arthritis Rheum 1988;31(3):315–24.
5. Steinbroker O, Traeger GH, Batterman RC. Therapeutic criteria in rheumatoid arthritis. JAMA 1949;140:659–62.
6. Sharp J, Lidsky M, Collins L, et al. Methods of scoring the progression of radiologic changes in rheumatoid arthritis. Arthritis Rheum 1971;14(6):706–20.

7. Larsen A, Knut Dale, Eek M. Radiographic evaluation of rheumatoid arthritis and related conditions by standard reference films. Acta Radiol Diagn 1977;18: 481–91.

8. Rau R, Wassenberg S, Herborn G, et al. A new method of scoring radiographic changes in rheumatoid arthritis. J Rheumatol 1998;25(11):2094–107.

9. Ostergaard M, Pedersen S, Dohn U. Imaging in rheumatoid arthritis—status and recent advances for magnetic resonance imaging, ultrasonography, computed tomography, and conventional radiography. Best Pract Res Clin Rheumatol 2008;22(6):1019–44.

10. Hetland M, Ejbjerg B, Horslev-Petersen K, et al. MRI bone edema is the strongest predictor of subsequent radiographic progression in early-rheumatoid arthritis. Results from a 2-year randomized controlled trial (CIMESTRA). Ann Rheum Dis 2009;68:384–90.

11. Haavardsholm E, Boyesen P, Ostergaard M, et al. Magnetic resonance imaging findings in 84 patients with early rheumatoid arthritis: bone marrow edema predicts erosive progression. Ann Rheum Dis 2008;67:794–800.

12. Boesen M, Ostergaard M, Cimmino M, et al. MRI quantification of rheumatoid arthritis: current knowledge and future prospectives. Eur J Radiol 2009;71(2): 189–96.

13. Freestone J, Bird P, Conaghan P. The role of MRI in rheumatoid arthritis: research and clinical issues. Curr Opin Rheumatol 2009;21:95–101.

14. Wakefield R, D'Agostino MA, Iagnocco A, et al. The OMERACT Ultrasound Group: status of current activities and research directions. J Rheumatol 2007; 34(4):848–51.

15. Lopez-Ben R. Rheumatoid arthritis: ultrasound assessment of synovitis and erosions. Ultrasound Clin 2007;2(4):727–36.

16. Wakefield R, Gibbon W, Conaghan P, et al. The value of sonography in the detection of bone erosions in patients with rheumatoid arthritis. Arthritis Rheum 2000; 43(12):2762–70.

17. Polster J, Winalski CS, Sundaram M, et al. Rheumatoid arthritis: evaluation with contrast-enhanced CT with digital bone masking. Radiology 2009;252(1):225–31.

Clinical Manifestations and Treatment of the Pediatric Rheumatoid Patient

Lawrence Haber, MD[a],*, Erika Womack, MS[a],
Catherine Zimmerman, MD[b], Joshua Hughes, BA[c]

KEYWORDS

• Ankle • Arthritis • Foot • Juvenile • Manifestations • Treatment

The management goal of juvenile rheumatoid arthritis (JRA) is to achieve early diagnosis and treatment so that arthritis can be resolved at an early stage, which avoids long-term damage and provides a good outcome of the affected inflammatory joints. This article describes presentation, classification, evaluation, and treatment of JRA as it relates to the foot and ankle. Because the course of JRA is complex and the optimal management is highly variable in each patient, this article can only offer recommendations. Actual treatment should be individualized to meet the conditions of each patient.

JRA is a chronic autoimmune inflammatory joint condition affecting children up to 16 years of age. Chronic inflammation of synovial membranes (synovitis) and articular structures can deteriorate synovial joints to the point of deformity and permanent joint dysfunction. Mode of onset and clinical features are varied. Classification is important in guiding treatment and is outlined in this article. Treatment is in accordance with the type of JRA and with individual manifestations, such as the onset, severity of disease, and prognostic measures. Some children may do well with conservative treatment. Others at risk for irreversible joint damage and poor functional outcome require a more aggressive therapy, however, to minimize morbidity and maximize normal growth and development.[1]

[a] Department of Orthopaedic Surgery, University of Mississippi Medical Center, 2500 North State Street, Jackson, MS 39216, USA
[b] Department of Pediatrics, University of Mississippi Medical Center, 2500 North State Street, Jackson, MS 39216, USA
[c] School of Medicine, University of Mississippi Medical Center, 2500 North State Street, Jackson, MS 39216, USA
* Corresponding author.
E-mail address: lhaber@orthopedics.umsmed.edu

Clin Podiatr Med Surg 27 (2010) 219–233
doi:10.1016/j.cpm.2009.12.006
0891-8422/10/$ – see front matter © 2010 Elsevier Inc. All rights reserved.

podiatric.theclinics.com

CLASSIFICATION OF JRA

The American College of Rheumatology (ACR) classifies JRA into three subgroups: (1) systemic, (2) pauciarticular, and (3) polyarticular arthritis. These subgroups are primarily based on the number of joints involved and associated symptoms. The European League Against Rheumatism classification, which uses the term "juvenile chronic arthritis," has a separate classification. Because of the discrepancies between the ACR and European League Against Rheumatism classifications, a task force was created by the pediatric standing Committee of the International League of Associations for Rheumatology. This task force proposed "juvenile idiopathic arthritis" as the unifying term that refers to a group of disorders characterized by chronic arthritis in childhood with onset before 16 years of age.[2–7] Both terms "JRA" and "juvenile idiopathic arthritis," however, are used throughout literature. For clarity, this article uses JRA as initially proposed by the ACR.

SIGNIFICANCE

Although arthritic indispositions in children are frequent, the incidence and prevalence of JRA is low. JRA, the most common rheumatic disorder in childhood, has an estimated worldwide prevalence of 0.07 to 4.01 per 1000 children[8] and 5 to 150 per 100,000 children (70,000–250,000 cases reported) in the United States population.[9–11] In general, girls are affected more than boys. Oligoarthritis accounts for most JRA cases (24%–58%) with a 4:1 female/male ratio.[12,13] Polyarthritis (rheumatoid factor [RF]-negative) accounts for 10% to 28% of all rheumatoid arthritis cases in children and affects mostly girls (3:1). Polyarthritis (RF-positive) is the least common, accounting for less than 10% of all JRA cases, and overwhelmingly affects girls over boys (9:1).[12] Systemic arthritis accounts for 2% to 20% of all JRA cases affecting boys as often as girls.[12–14]

JRA SUBSETS
Pauciarticular JRA

Pauciarticular (oligoarticular [oJRA]) JRA is the most common subset and is defined as having four or fewer joints affected for at least 6 months. Half of the patients present with complaints of only one affected joint (monoarticular).[15,16] Signs may include pain; gait abnormalities; stiffness; or warm, swollen joints. Other causes must be excluded. The time of onset is most often before 5 years of age. As a result of a positive testing of antinuclear antibody (ANA), patients of this subset have a greater risk of developing uveitis.[17]

Manifestations of oJRA

Large joint most commonly affected is the knee followed by the ankle and wrist.[17,18] In one study, ankle involvement with or without wrist involvement, symmetric disease, and laboratory evidence of inflammation (increased erythrocyte sedimentation rate [ESR]) within the first 6 months of illness indicated association with higher risk of extended disease course.[19] Extended pauciarticular JRA with additional joint involvement after the first 6 months (more than four joints ultimately affected over time) can occur and usually has a worse prognosis.

Patients of this subset do not experience systemic symptoms (except uveitis) and often do not complain of pain. Uveitis is a serious complication and occurs in 30% to 50% of patients.[20] The inflammation of the eye can lead to scarring of the iris (synechiae); corneal clouding; cataracts; glaucoma; and partial or total vision impairment.[21] All patients must be referred to an ophthalmologist for frequent evaluation. The risk of uveitis is greatest in children less than 6 years of age with positive ANA and usually requires more frequent eye examinations.[22] Most children with JRA who develop uveitis achieve good visual outcome despite uveitic complications.[23]

Another significant complication of oJRA is leg length discrepancy. Inflammation of the joint leads to hyperemia, increasing blood flow to the affected extremity and the activity of the physis near the joint. With monoarticular joint inflammation, alterations in activity of the physis can cause asymmetric growth; this occurs most often in the knee and ankle. In a retrospective study of children with pauciarticular and monoarticular arthritis, overgrowth of the involved extremity occurred in children who developed disease before the age of 9 with most having overgrowth before the age of 5. Those who developed the disease after the age of 9, however, had rapid premature epiphyseal plate closure resulting in shortening of the affected limb.[24] Etiology for rapid epiphyseal growth plate closure is unknown. The asymmetric and monoarticular nature of pauciarticular disease makes these discrepancies more pronounced.[25]

Polyarticular JRA

Initially, polyarticular JRA only involves one joint. As the disorder progresses, multiple joints are involved. Polyarticular JRA is defined as having more than four affected joints during the initial 6 months of disease with limitation of motion, tenderness or pain, or joint warmth.[18] Polyarticular arthritis may be further characterized according to the presence or absence of RF.

Manifestations of Polyarticular JRA

Clinical manifestations of polyarticular JRA are highly variable presenting with any combination of anemia, anorexia, growth retardation, and osteopenia. Patterns of presentation are based on age of onset. Similar to pauciarticular JRA, larger joints are commonly affected. Small joints of the feet and hands can be involved and may present as dactylitis (swelling and inflammation of the digits). Ankle and hindfoot involvement in persistent polyarthritis is common depending, to some extent, on the age of presentation. If there is a rapid increase (days to weeks) in the number of involved joints, reactive arthritis (postinfectious) should be considered. Systemic symptoms can be present but are usually mild in comparison with systemic onset.

SYSTEMIC JRA

Systemic JRA (sJRA) is defined as having any joint involvement with associated systemic features, including fever of at least 2 weeks and at least one of the following: an evanescent rash, lymphadenopathy, hepatosplenomegaly, or serositis.[18] Children with sJRA often have delayed growth, osteopenia, anemia, leukocytosis, thrombocytosis, and elevated acute-phase reactants. Most systemic features resolve when fever diminishes. Unlike with pauciarticular JRA in which asymmetry of disease leads to discrepancies of growth, sJRA patients may suffer from overall growth retardation because of symmetry of disease.

Manifestations of sJRA

Most typical features of sJRA include fever, arthritis, rash, and lymphadenopathy, which can all precede arthritis and positive laboratory findings by months to years. Fever occurs in many patients with varied patterns. Joint pain is frequently more pronounced when fever is elevated. Systemic JRA often affects the knees, wrists, and ankles. Ankle and tarsal joints, in addition to metatarsophalangeal joint involvement in persistent sJRA, may become damaged, often in an asymmetric fashion. This may cause a small foot with some toe elongation and others shortened.

Most children present with more than one involved joint. Because these children seem ill, their symptoms can be mistaken for malignancy on initial presentation. Acute lymphocytic leukemia may initially be misdiagnosed as JRA.[17,26] Acute lymphocytic leukemia can often present with joint pain and swelling well before peripheral blasts appear in the blood smear. Strong consideration of underlying leukemia as the cause of bone-joint complaints is suggested in children with concurrent changes on complete blood count (CBC [low red blood cell count, low to normal platelet count]) with history of nighttime pain.[27] This holds true for all patients that initially present with rheumatic complaints, with or without fever, in which the features of back pain, night sweats, bruising, and severe pain are atypical.[27–29]

PROGNOSIS (OF ALL SUBSETS)

Patients with JRA are thought to have an overall positive outcome; many go into remission and have no signs of limitation in adulthood. In 10-year follow-up studies, 33% to 50% of patients with JRA achieved remission.[30,31] Even so, morbidity persisting into adulthood is one of the greatest problems patients may face. More than 10% to 30% of people with childhood-onset arthritis have significant functional limitations after 10 or more years.[32,33]

Both the course and prognosis of JRA are variable and depend on the subset of JRA present in the patient. In particular, the long-term prognosis for children with polyarticular JRA is highly variable and hard to predict. Children with polyarticular JRA often seem to improve, then worsen repeatedly over a period of years. In patients with recurrences despite therapy, the risk of functional impairment is significant.[17] Polyarthritis RF-positive patients usually peak in late childhood or adolescence. In older females with positive RF, rapid involvement of joint can occur over a few months along with early erosion and rheumatoid nodules. This group is at risk for having a chronic course into adulthood.[34] The prognosis for oligoarthritis JRA varies. For most patients the disease is milder compared with other subtypes and the overall outcome is good.[35] Prognosis for systemic JRA is determined by the severity of the arthritis and systemic features. Most patients with sJRA initially seem well after 6 months and have resolution of arthritis. Others may have recurrence of arthritis years later and the remaining continue to be ill for prolonged periods of time.[17]

Patients with JRA that causes significant functional limitations most often have continuation of active disease. Concerning function, systemic arthritis followed by RF-positive polyarticular arthritis has the worst prognosis.[33,36] Clinicians should remember that despite efforts to establish trends with different subsets of JRA, presentation of symptoms and course and prognosis of the disease can be highly variable.[4,5,7] If a basic medical program is not enough, progression of disease into adulthood and even young adolescence may require aggressive intervention to regain or preserve function.

ASSESSMENT

Early evaluation of the patient is essential to increase the likelihood of a good outcome. JRA is a diagnosis of exclusion. Other causes of joint pain and swelling that must be ruled out include trauma, infection, toxic synovitis, spinal disorders, malignant or benign bone lesion, and other systemic rheumatologic diseases.

Diagnosis cannot be confirmed with complete confidence without a detailed patient history, physical examination, and laboratory testing.

Patient History

A detailed history is essential to separate benign from pathologic etiologies. This should include the presence of antecedent infection or trauma. Documentation of specific joint involvement, length and type of involvement, gait changes, and presence of stiffness is critical. Concerning pain and swelling, location and number of joints involved, frequency, duration, pattern, and exacerbating factors are important. Analysis of the associated warmth and redness of a joint is also important. Pain and morning stiffness, although subjective and not solely reliable to the degree of inflammation present, must be assessed.[37] Pain and stiffness is usually worse in the mornings, improves with movement and activity, and worsens with inactivity.

In addition, a thorough review of systems that focuses on fever, rash, weight loss, abdominal pain, and ocular abnormalities is necessary. The fever trend associated with systemic JRA usually spikes in the evenings and returns to normal by morning. Family history is important to search for diseases associated with JRA, such as celiac disease, inflammatory bowel disease, psoriasis, and uveitis. Although uveitis should be screened for, it is usually not symptomatic early in the course of JRA.

Physical Examination

An overview of the patient's medical history should be followed by a complete physical examination. In addition to the physical examination, force distribution under the foot has been measured in children with ankle and hindfoot involvement to assess the effect of deformities on foot function compared with normal children. General inspection of patient, growth parameters, vital signs, and general observation of simple physical maneuvers by way of pediatric gait-arms-legs-spine examination should be assessed. The pediatric gait-arms-legs-spine is a simple, fast, and valid way to assess for normal or abnormal joint movement in pediatric patients. Adult gait-arms-legs-spine should not be used because it has been shown to miss important foot and ankle abnormalities.[38]

A focused examination of affected and unaffected joints should include gross examination; palpation of joints, bones, and points of insertion of tendons and ligaments; range of motion; and strength. Most often one joint is involved in arthritis (monoarticular) and progression to other joints can occur over a course of weeks to months. Small outpunching of synovium may be appreciated around the ankle along with tenosynovitis. Tenosynovitis most often occurs on the extensor sheaths over the dorsum of foot and the peroneus longus and brevis tendons around the ankle. Posterior tibial tendonitis has been documented as a presenting feature (unpublished data, 2009). Firm, mobile, and nontender and rheumatoid nodules can occur over the Achilles tendon.[4]

Diagnostics and Laboratory Testing

Joint aspiration and synovial fluid examination are useful to rule out other causes of arthropathy. Moreover, it can aid in the diagnosis of JRA. White blood cell (WBC) count can be beneficial in helping to distinguish JRA from an infected joint. Usually, a WBC count greater than 40,000 cells/mm^3 is associated with infectious arthritis. Patients with JRA can have a much higher WBC, however, up to 100,000 cell/mm^3. High WBC is not a diagnostic for an infectious joint.[39,40] The principle cellular components of joint aspiration analysis in children with JRA are polymorphonuclear neutrophils, most often seen in polyarticular and systemic JRA; mononuclear cells are often dominant in pauciarticular JRA.[41] Overall, high or low cell count has not been shown to correlate with disease activity.[4] Protein, glucose, and lactate of synovial fluid offer limited diagnostic value.[41] Hyaluronic acid and chondroitin sulfates levels are lower in synovial fluid when compared with controls.[42] Recent research has evaluated specific protein biomarkers found in the synovial fluid of children with recurrent inflammation. The expression of these proteins may help identify children who are at higher risk for recurrent inflammation and progression of disease.[43,44]

Laboratory studies have an important role in excluding specific causes of JRA. CBC, blood chemistries, C-reactive protein (CRP), ESR, lactate dehydrogenase, creatine kinase, and routine urinalysis[34] can aid in ruling out other causes of joint pain and swelling, including infection and malignancy. Testing for Lyme disease (endemic areas)[45] and group A streptococcus may be beneficial. ANA, RF, and HLA-B27 marker is warranted in suspected cases. These markers are often negative in children with JRA resulting in a high false-negative rate.[4,29] In monoarthritis and mild cases of oligoarticular JRA, the ESR and CRP are often mildly elevated. In more severe cases of oJRA, the ESR and CRP are raised. There is also no presence of RF in oJRA; ANA is frequently positive.[17] Laboratory findings for polyarticular RF-negative JRA are often associated with a positive ANA and an absence of RF. RF-positive polyarticular JRA, as its name implies, is positive for the RF and is usually positive for HLA-DR4.[46] Laboratory findings for systemic JRA include positive markers for inflammation including elevated CRP and ESR, elevated median WBC count, and low median hemoglobin.[28] Macrophage activation syndrome is almost exclusively seen in systemic JRA and is a life-threatening complication that involves multiple organs. The syndrome may be precipitated by viral infections.[47]

Radiographs are an important way of determining function, development, and involvement of the foot and ankle. When able, standing films should be done. Ankle films should include anterior-posterior, lateral, and mortise views of the ankle. Anterior-posterior, lateral, and oblique views of the foot are important for foot symptoms. Lateral radiograph of the foot and ankle when standing in full dorsiflexion and plantar flexion can be useful to document the degree of motion. Early changes that can be appreciated by simple films include periarticular soft tissue swelling and widening of the joint space with periosteal new bone apposition involving metatarsals. Later radiographic findings can reveal narrowing of joint spaces in ankle and subtalar joints with subluxation and ankylosis in smaller joints of the feet.[48] Boney erosion may take years to become visible on simple imaging.

In joints that are difficult to evaluate for effusion, more sensitive imaging can obtain accurate identification of the anatomic damage caused by inflammatory processes.[49] MRI is the most useful to identify tenosynovitis, synovitis, enthesitis, bone erosions,[48] or small joint involvement. It also avoids radiation risks. Diagnostic imaging, such as radionuclide bone scans and CT, can sometimes help when etiology is still unclear. Although the role of a CT scan is limited, it can be helpful to reveal smaller areas with arthritic irregularities. CT is unlikely to be useful in small children because of lack of ossification. Because CT involves significant radiation exposure, use of the procedure should be carefully considered in children. Ultrasonography is an inexpensive and valuable diagnostic imaging technique that can demonstrate both inflammatory and destructive changes and effusions.[50,51] Unfortunately, the lack of an experienced ultrasonagrapher limits its application in most institutions.

Foot and Ankle Involvement in JRA

A number of deformities can occur in the rheumatic arthritic child. Authors have documented that the lower extremity of a patient with JRA may present with pain, joint effusion, synovitis, deformity, stiffness, and limited joint range of motion.[52,53] Foot and ankle problems have commonly been reported in JRA.[54,55] Severe inflammation can occur in the forefoot, hindfoot, and ankle. In all JRA cases, inflammation of the ankle, tarsal, and metatarsophalangeal joints is found in 51% to 59%, 1% to 13%, and 49% to 68%, respectively.[56] Foot and ankle complications of the JRA patient are familiar, but relatively disregarded.[57]

The arthritic forefoot, which consists of the interphalangeal and metatarsophalangeal joints, creates deforming biomechanical forces that can act on the hindfoot and ankle and ultimately the rest of the body.[55] The interphalangeal or metatarsophalangeal joint may induce clawing of the toes. In addition to clawing, the interphalangeal joints may become dislocated or ankylosed. Pain and swelling may elicit muscle contractions and eventual phalangeal joint flexion deformities may occur.[55] Hallux valgus frequently develops; hallux rigidus may also occur (**Fig. 1**). The hindfoot controls varus and valgus or supination and pronation. Significant pronation of the foot, a frequent finding in JRA patients, occurs when synovitis stretches the capsule and ligaments of the subtalar and talonavicular joints causing subsequent calcaneal pressure. Varus deformity can also occur because of synovitis, usually as a compensatory measure to prevent pressure on the metatarsophalangeal and subtalar joints during ambulation.[58]

Ankle involvement in JRA is the second most common after the knee.[59] The ankle joint allows dorsiflexion and plantarflexion. The loss of dorsiflexion because of synovitis can impede ambulation.[56] The loss of plantar flexion, although less common, can occur and cause gait distortion. To sustain function and minimize deformity, early recognition of these signs and application of effective JRA therapy are vital.

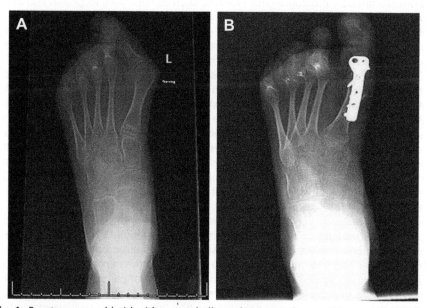

Fig. 1. Fourteen-year-old girl with severe hallux valgus secondary to JRA treated with first MTP joint fusion. (*A*) Preoperative radiograph. (*B*) Postoperative radiograph of MTP joint fusion.

TREATMENT OF JRA
General Treatment

Treatment and management of JRA in the foot and ankle include controlling inflammation, relieving and managing pain, preventing or controlling joint damage, increasing range of motion, and achieving long-term remission. To achieve management, treatment for foot and ankle disease in JRA has focused on pharmacologic therapy, intra-articularcorticosteroid injections, physical therapy, and orthoses. When most conservative measures fail, surgery may be necessary to resolve synovitis and correct or maintain foot posture and function.

Pharmacologic Therapy

Pharmacological therapy is critical for the management of JRA. Coordination with a rheumatologist is essential to properly treat any child with this disorder. The primary principles of pharmacological therapy in JRAs are to suppress inflammation, decrease or eliminate pain, and promote and maintain remission with the least possible adverse effects. Medications are individualized to the specific needs of each patient depending on the severity of his or her subtype and prior response to other drugs. Pharmacological management of JRA has been improved with the earlier use of nonsteroidal anti-inflammatory drugs (NSAIDs), intra-articular corticosteroid injections, and disease-modifying anti-rheumatic drugs (DMARDs) with the inclusion of tumor necrosis factor (TNF) inhibiting agents. The progressive development of these drugs has improved treatment options for the pediatric patient. Functional outcomes seem to have improved as a result.[58,60]

NSAIDs are typically the first-line of therapy. NSAIDs contribute symptomatic relief by providing an analgesia and anti-inflammatory effect which are controlled by the inhibition of the enzyme, cyclooxygenase (COX); NSAIDs prevent the production of the proinflammatory prostaglandins. NSAIDs, such as naproxen, ibuprofen and celecoxib, are commonly used. Most NSAIDs are well tolerated with few side effects in children. Unfortunately, nearly two-thirds of children with juvenile arthritis do not respond well to NSAIDs or have inadequate treatment.[61] When response is poor, these patients must resort to alternative pharmacologic interventions.

DMARDs, a second-line therapy, are often used to treat patients with JRA who do not respond effectively to NSAIDs. Early initiation of aggressive therapy by introducing DMARDs provides a better prognosis.[62] Methotrexate is the most commonly used DMARD for treatment of persistent juvenile arthritis. Methotrexate may decrease the severity of pain, improve ranges of motion, and decrease the ESR. This drug can also be used to decrease the severity of uveitis in children with JRA.[63] When patients inadequately respond to methotrexate, etanercept (Enbrel) and adalimumab (Humira), TNF blocking DMARDs can be used in conjunction with methotrexate.[64,65] DMARDs are usually well tolerated; the most frequent adverse effects tend to affect blood cells, liver, and skin.

Intra-articular steroid injections are also used for treatment in children in conjunction with other medications or in children who have not responded to other medications. Prior to injections, arthritis due to Lyme disease must be ruled out in endemic areas. Intra-articular corticosteroid injections have proven effective in controlling synovitis in JRA and may help induce remission.[66] In monoarticular or pauciarticular JRA, injections may lead to complete resolution of symptoms obviating the need for regular systemic therapy. In children with polyarticular JRA, the strategy of multiple intra-articular injections to induce disease remission while simultaneously initiating therapy with disease-modifying agents has been proposed.[66] Intra-articular hydrocortisone injected into inflamed interphalangeal and metatarsophalangeal joints reduces claw-ing of the toes and provides relief. Triamcinolone hexacetonide is a commonly used intra-articular corticosteroid injection and often controls inflammation. Used within 2 months of diagnosis and, if necessary, repeatedly, intra-articular steroids have been shown to prevent the well-recognized complication of leg-length discrepancy in pau-ciarticular JRA and polyarticular JRA.[67] Despite pharmacologic advances, ankle- and foot-related impairment and disability persists in some children with JRA.

Surgical Intervention in JRA

The ability of current medical treatment to control inflammation and subsequent joint damage limits the role of foot and ankle surgery in most children with JRA; however, in severe cases, surgery may be necessary. In a long-term study associated with juvenile arthritis, 22% of study participants have been subjected to surgery.[32] The aims of surgery, in particularly in the foot and ankle of patients with JRA, are to maintain or improve joint function, relieve disabling pain, or restore function when conservative measures have failed. Rheumatologists and foot and ankle surgeons confront distinct challenges when treating JRA patients who need surgery because of the complexity of the deformity caused by soft tissue contractures, small bone size, and concerns about future growth. The main complications after foot and ankle surgery include skin slough, infection, nonunion, and malunion. Complication rates are increased, in part, because of the steroids and other medications used. The decision to perform surgery must be made by an interdisciplinary team, including a rheumatologist, and based on an analysis of the risks and benefits for each child.

Synovectomy

Deterioration of cartilage, excessive growth of the synovium, and inflammation even-tually leads to damage of the joint surface causing stiffness and pain in the JRA patient. Synovectomy may be warranted in children when the arthritic ankle joint is deficient to conservative therapies. Indications for synovectomy are persistent syno-vitis nonresponsive to other conventional therapies (**Fig. 2**). Synovectomy surgery may be performed for the relief of pain, edema, and restricted range of motion. Early syn-ovectomy might prevent further joint damage and diminish pain, inflammation, and swelling in the effected joint (**Fig. 3**A); however, the range of motion is unlikely to improve and may worsen.[68,69] The results of synovectomy depend on good postop-erative therapy to ensure maximum benefit. Benefits generally seem to outweigh the disadvantages of performing synovectomy in growing children with JRA unresponsive to other treatment modalities.[68] Synovectomies can be performed as an open surgical procedure or arthroscopically.[70] This treatment is most relevant for the ankle.

Soft Tissue Release

Tendons and joint capsules associated with the foot and ankle may become inflamed causing considerable pain, stiffness, and deformity. Release or lengthening may be indicated if soft tissue, such as a tendon or joint capsule, becomes tight and causes functional problems. These procedures should not be done during active disease. Only deformities that are passively correctable can be treated with soft tissue proce-dures alone. Releases and lengthenings can alleviate joint contractures, increase the total range of movement, and relieve pain in a child with JRA.[71] Resistant equinus of the ankle may be corrected by Achilles tendon lengthening and capsulotomies of the ankle and subtalar joints.[72] Soft tissue release may also be indicated for deformities, such as varus of the hindfoot.[73] This deformity may be corrected by performing a post-eromedial release with tendon transfers as needed.[72]

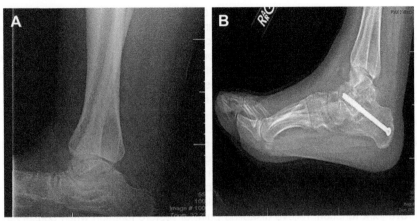

Fig. 2. A 15-year-old girl with juvenile arthritis and involvement of the right ankle caused by progressive, severe, and painful subluxation. (*A*) Preoperative radiographs with two views of the right ankle show soft tissue swelling and effusion at the level of the ankle. (*B*) Postoperative radiograph of subtalar arthrodesis of the right foot showed a screw transfixing the talocalcaneal joint, with an overlying cast. The surgical intervention included right posterior tibial tendon, flexor digitorum, and posterior ankle synovectomy, right subtalar arthrodesis with iliac crest graft and excision of accessory navicular.

ARTHRODESIS

Arthrodesis may be proposed for the treatment of persistent joint damage of the foot and ankle caused by synovitis in patients with JRA as a result of failure of conservative therapy (see **Fig. 2**). Fusions can be used to correct rigid deformity and decrease pain in an inflamed joint. When performing fusions, one must respect the role of growth centers and physes and avoid these procedures in young children. In some patients, the subtalar or talonavicular joint may be the only joint in the hindfoot with significant involvement. For these patients, a single arthrodesis is recommended.[3] Although ankle arthrodesis provides pain relief and acceptable function in most patients, it has the disadvantage of producing an immobile joint, or worsening pre-existing degenerative changes. Correction of a deformity without arthrodesis is preferable.[74] An immobile ankle joint increases stress on the subtalar and midtarsal joints causing the loss of the compensatory mechanisms in the foot required for comfortable gait.[75]

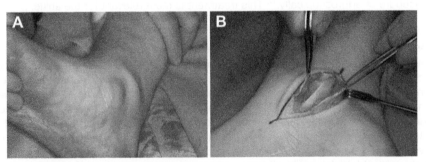

Fig. 3. JRA patient presenting as posterior tendon synovitis. (*A*) Preoperative photo of an ankle presenting with medial swelling. (*B*) Intraoperative photo of the posterior tendon synovectomy, in part performed for diagnosis.

Once children reach the age of 12 to 14 and the disability persists despite conservative measures, fixed deformities of the hindfoot may best be corrected by performing a triple arthrodesis.[72] A triple arthrodesis eliminates the subtalar and transverse tarsal joint motion, increasing stress on the ankle and the midtarsal joints distal to the fusion site.[3,76]

Some complications of arthrodesis include delayed wound healing; infection; nonunion of the ankle; malunion of the ankle joint with the foot; and neuropathy. Some other problems common after ankle arthrodesis for JRA include excessive plantar flexion, which may cause knee discomfort; excessive dorsiflexion, which may cause stress on the heel; varus deformity, which results in subtalar joint instability; and excessive valgus causing stress on the medial aspect of the knee joint.[76,77] Although arthrodesis provides a more reliable long-term function and remains the standard of treatment, total ankle arthroplasty has been proposed as an alternative to ankle arthrodesis in severe ankle involvement.

Total Joint Replacement (Arthroplasty)

There are few reports of ankle arthroplasty specifically in patients with JRA. Total ankle replacement is indicated when cartilage damage to the joint causes deteriorating function and persistent debilitating pain nonresponsive to conservative measures.[34] The difficulties of arthroplasty are largely caused by poor bone quality from the associated deformities and malunion of the ankle and subtalar joints. Advantages of performing an arthroplasty, as an alternative to ankle arthrodesis, include preservation of some ankle joint motion with a more normal gait leading to less stress on adjacent joints.[1]

Physical Therapy

Physical therapy is vital in the care of children with JRA involving the foot and ankle. Therapists assess restrictions in joint movement and joint function and provide plans for long-term rehabilitation programs. Physical therapists also prescribe and monitor exercise and splinting programs for families to perform with the child at home; these programs improve or maintain joint motion and muscle strength and help avoid muscle contractures.[34] Exercise maintains strength and range of motion, encourages growth, and helps prevent deformity. Weight bearing exercises might be difficult for the JRA patient with foot and ankle problems; therefore, swimming and cycling are advantageous activities that provide muscle strengthening and increase range of motion.[78] For children with severe flexion contractures, a dynamic tension splint or serial casting can be used to correct the contracture.[79] Orthotics are often used for ankle or subtalar arthritis for foot deformities to decrease pain when walking, improve gait, provide arch support for flatfoot, and minimize pressure on metatarsal heads to prevent the formation of callus or subluxation of the toes.[34] The ankle-foot arthosis also may be used to correct hindfoot and forefoot malalignment by reducing persistent peroneal or posterior tibialis spasm or marked muscle imbalance when patients are nonresponsive to a heel-cup orthosis.[34] Patients with leg length discrepancy occasionally need shoe lifts in the leg that has suffered growth retardation.

SUMMARY

The course of JRA is variable, unpredictable, and unique in each patient. The efforts of a team of health care professionals, including a rheumatologist, should be performed in concert in a coordinated system of management that is individualized to meet the needs of each patient. To provide optimum foot and ankle care, it is essential to monitor disease activity and early joint destruction.[80] The therapeutic program must also screen and provide appropriate treatment for other symptomatic problems, such as uveitis. Treatment goals for JRA are to relieve pain and prevent contractures and deformities by achieving early and complete suppression of inflammation without treatment toxicity while maintaining power, joint range of movement, and function through active physical therapy and if necessary surgery. A careful and considerate approach to the surgical management of JRA can lead to improved function and significant pain relief for children with the affliction. Although treatment of JRA is complex and challenging, early diagnosis and comprehensive therapy can diminish joint deformity and maximize normal growth and development.

REFERENCES

1. Klepper SE. Juvenile idiopathic arthritis. In: Tecklin JS, editor. Pediatric physical therapy. 4th edition. Philadelphia: Lippincott Williams and Wilkins; 2008. p. 487–532.
2. Petty RE, Southwood TR, Manners P, et al. International League of Associations for Rheumatology classification of juvenile idiopathic arthritis. J Rheumatol 2004;31(2):390–2.
3. Petty RE, Southwood TR, Baum J, et al. Revision of the proposed classification criteria for juvenile idiopathic arthritis. J Rheumatol 1998;25:1991–4.
4. Cassidy JT, Petty RE. Juvenile rheumatoid arthritis. In: Cassidy JT, Petty RE, editors. Textbook of pediatric rheumatology. 4th edition. Philadelphia: W.B. Sanders Company; 2001. p. 218–321.
5. Brewer EJ, Bass JC, Cassidy TJ, et al. Criteria for the classification of juvenile rheumatoid arthritis. Bull Rheum Dis 1973;23:712–9.
6. Weiss JE, Ilowite NT. Juvenile idiopathic arthritis. Rheum Dis Clin North Am 2007; 33(3):441–70.
7. Schneider R, Passo MH. Juvenile rheumatoid arthritis. Rheum Dis Clin North Am 2002;28(3):503–30.
8. Manners PJ, Bower C. Worldwide prevalence of juvenile arthritis: why does it vary so much? J Rheumatol 2002;29:1520–30.
9. Andersson GB. Epidemiology. Baillieres Clin Rheumatol 1998;12(2):191–208.
10. Oen KG, Cheang M. Epidemiology of chronic arthritis in childhood. Semin Arthritis Rheum 1996;26:575–91.
11. Andersson GB. Juvenile arthritis: who gets it, where and when? A review of current data on incidence and prevalence. Clin Exp Rheumatol 1999;17(5): 347–79.
12. Hofer M, Southwood TR. Classification of childhood arthritis. Best Pract Res Clin Rheumatol 2002;16:379–96.
13. Malleson PN, Fung MY, Rosenburg AM. The incidence of pediatric rheumatic diseased: results from the Canadian Pediatric Rheumatology Association. J Rheumatol 1996;23:1981–7.
14. Hendry G, Gardner-Medwin J, Watt GF. A survey of foot problems in juvenile idiopathic arthritis. Musculoskeletal Care 2008;6(4):221–32.
15. Cassidy JT, Brody GI, Martel W. Monoarticular juvenile rheumatoid arthritis. J Pediatr 1967;70:867–75.
16. Bywater EGL, Ansell BM. Monoarticular arthritis in children. Ann Rheum Dis 1965; 24(2):116–22.
17. Lehman TJ. Juvenile rheumatoid arthritis. In: Saulco TP, editor. Surgical treatment of rheumatoid arthritis. St. Louis (MO): Mosby-Yearbook Inc; 1992. p. 11–21.

18. Southwood TR, Woo P. Juvenile chronic arthritis. Best Pract Res Clin Rheumatol 1995;9(2):331–53.
19. Al Matar MJ, Petty RE, Tucker LB, et al. The early pattern of joint involvement predicts disease progression in children with oligoarticular (pauciarticular) juvenile rheumatoid arthritis. Arthritis Rheum 2002;46(10):2708–15.
20. Saurenmann RK, Levin AV, Feldman BM, et al. Prevalence, risk factors and outcome of uveitis in juvenile idiopathic arthritis: a longterm follow-up study. Arthritis Rheum 2007;56(2):647–57.
21. Kotaniemi K, Savolainen A, Karma A. Recent advances in uveitis of juvenile idiopathic arthritis. Surv Ophthalmol 2003;48(5):489–502.
22. Cassidy J, Kivlin J, Lindsley C, et al. Ophthalmologic examinations in children with juvenile rheumatoid arthritis. Pediatrics 2006;117(5):1843–5.
23. Sabri K, Saurenmann RK, Silverman ED, et al. Course, complications, and outcome of juvenile arthritis-related uveitis. J AAPOS 2008;12(6):537–8.
24. Simon S, Whiffen J, Shapiro F. Leg-length discrepancies in monoarticular and pauciarticular juvenile rheumatoid arthritis. J Bone Joint Surg Am 1981;63(2):209–15.
25. Vostrejs M, Hollister JR. Muscle atrophy and leg length discrepancy in pauciarticular juvenile arthritis. Am J Dis Child 1988;142:343–5.
26. Murray MJ, Tang T, Ryder C, et al. Childhood leukaemia masquerading as juvenile idiopathic arthritis. BMJ 2004;329:959–61.
27. Jones OY, Spencer HC, Bowyer SL, et al. A multicenter case control study in predictive factors distinguishing childhood leukemia from juvenile rheumatoid arthritis. Pediatrics 2006;117(5):840–4.
28. Behrens EM, Beukelman T, Gallo L, et al. Evaluation of the presentation of systemic onset juvenile rheumatoid arthritis: data from the Pennsylvania Systemic Onset Juvenile Arthritis Registry(PASOJAR). J Rheumatol 2008;35(2):343–8.
29. Cabral DA, Tucker LB. Malignancies in children who initially present with rheumatic complaints. J Pediatr 1999;134(1):53–7.
30. Fantini F, Gerloni V, Gattinara M, et al. Remission in juvenile chronic arthritis: a cohort study of 683 consecutive cases with a mean 10 year followup. J Rheumatol 2003;30(3):579–84.
31. Minden K, Kiessling U, Listing J, et al. Prognosis of patients with juvenile chronic arthritis and juvenile spondyloarthropathy. J Rheumatol 2000;27(9):2256–63.
32. Zak M, Pedersen FK. Juvenile chronic arthritis into adulthood: a long-term follow-up study. Rheumatology (Oxford) 2000;39:198–204.
33. Ravelli A. Toward an understanding of the long-term outcome of juvenile idiopathic arthritis. Clin Exp Rheumatol 2004;22(3):271–5.
34. Hashkes PJ, Laxer RM. Juvenile idiopathic arthritis: treatment and assessment. In: Klippel JH, Stone JH, Crofford LJ, editors. Primer on the rheumatic diseases. 13th edition. New York: Springer; 2008. p. 154–62.
35. Adib N, Silman A, Thomson W. Outcome following onset of juvenile idiopathic inflammatory arthritis: I. frequency of different outcomes. Rheumatology (Oxford) 2005;44(8):995–1001.
36. Packman JC, Hall MA. Long-term follow-up of 246 adults with juvenile idiopathic arthritis: functional outcome. Rheumatology 2002;41:1428–35.
37. Ilowite NT, Walco GA, Pochaczevsky R. Assessment of pain in patients with juvenile rheumatoid arthritis: relation between pain intensity and degree of joint inflammation. Ann Rheum Dis 1992;51:343–6.
38. Foster HE, Kay LJ, Friswell M, et al. Musculoskeletal screening examination (pGALS) for school age children based on the adult GALS screen. Arthritis Rheum 2006;55(5):709–16.

39. Zuckner J, Baldassare AR, Chang F, et al. High synovial fluid leukocyte counts not associated with infectious arthritis. Arthritis Rheum 1977;20:270.

40. Baldassare AR, Chang F, Zuckner J. Markedly raised synovial fluid leukocyte counts not associated with infection arthritis in children. Ann Rheum Dis 1978; 37:404–9.

41. Kunnamo I, Pelkonen P. Routine analysis of synovial fluid cells is of value in the differential diagnosis of arthritis in children. J Rheumatol 1986;13(6):1076–80.

42. Spelling PF, Heise N, Toledo OM. Glycosaminoglycans in the synovial fluids of patients with juvenile rheumatoid arthritis. Clin Exp Rheumatol 1991;9:195–9.

43. Gibson DS, Blelock S, Curry J, et al. Comparative analysis of synovial fluid and plasma proteomes in juvenile arthritis: proteomic patterns of joint inflammation in early stage of disease. J Proteomics 2009;72(4):656–76.

44. Gibson DS, Blelock S, Curry J, et al. Proteomic analysis of recurrent joint inflammation in juvenile idiopathic arthritis. J Proteome Res 2006;5(8):1988–95.

45. Huppertz HI. Lyme disease in children. Curr Opin Rheumatol 2001;13(5):434–40.

46. Stastny P, Fink CW. Different HLA-D associations in adult and juvenile rheumatoid arthritis. J Clin Invest 1979;63:124–30.

47. Stephan JL, Kone Paut I, Galambrun C, et al. Reactive haemophagocytic syndrome in children with inflammatory disorders: a retrospective study of 24 patients. Rheumatology 2001;40(11):1285–92.

48. Babyn P, Doria AS. Radiologic investigation of rheumatic diseases. Pediatr Clin North Am 2005;52:373–411.

49. Grassi W, Salaffi F, Filippucci E. Ultrasound in Rheumatology. Best Pract Res Clin Rheumatol 2005;19(3):467–85.

50. Filippucci E, Farina A, Cervini C, et al. Juvenile chronic arthritis and imaging: comparison of different techniques. Reumatismo 2001;53:63–7.

51. Graeme TB. Imaging in juvenile arthritis. Curr Opin Rheumatol 2005;17:574–8.

52. Spraul G, Koenning G. A descriptive study of foot problems in children with juvenile rheumatoid arthritis. Arthritis Care Res 1994;7(3):144–50.

53. Schaller J, Wedgewood RJ. Juvenile rheumatoid arthritis: a review. Pediatrics 1972;50:940–53.

54. Foster HE, Eltringham MS, Kay LJ, et al. Delay in access to appropriate care for children presenting with musculoskeletal symptoms and ultimately diagnosed with juvenile idiopathic arthritis. Arthritis Rheum 2007;57(6):921–7.

55. Melvin JL, Atwood M. Juvenile rheumatoid arthritis. In: Melvin JL, editor. Rheumatic disease in the adult and child: occupational therapy and rehabilitation. 3rd edition. Philadelphia: F.A. Davis Company; 1989. p. 135–84.

56. Rothschild BM. Recognition and treatment of arthritis in children. Compr Ther 1999;25(6–7):347–59.

57. Hendry GJ, Turner DE, McColl J, et al. Protocol for the Foot in Juvenile Idiopathic Arthritis trial (FiJIA): a randomised controlled trial of an integrated foot care programme for foot problems in JIA. J Foot Ankle Res 2009;2:21.

58. Swann M. Management of lower limb deformities. In: Arden GP, Ansell BP, editors. Surgical management of juvenile chronic polyarthritis. New York: Grune & Stratton; 1978. p. 97–115.

59. Zimbler S, McVerr B, Levine P. Hemophilic arthropathy of the foot and ankle. Orthop Clin North Am 1976;7:985–7.

60. Murray KJ, Lovell DJ. Advanced therapy for juvenile arthritis. Best Pract Res Clin Rheumatol 2002;16(3):361–78.

61. Chikanza IC. Juvenile rheumatoid arthritis: therapeutic perspectives. Paediatr Drugs 2002;4(5):335–48.

62. Ilowite NT. Current treatment of juvenile rheumatoid arthritis. Pediatrics 2002; 109(1):109–15.
63. Giannini EH, Cawkwell GD. Drug treatment in children with juvenile rheumatoid arthritis: past, present, and future. Pediatr Clin North Am 1995;42:1099–125.
64. Weiss AH, Wallace CA, Sherry DD. Methotrexate for resistance chronic uveitis in children with juvenile rheumatoid arthritis. J Pediatr 1998;133:266.
65. Foeldvari I, Wierk A. Methotrexate is an effective treatment for chronic uveitis associated with juvenile idiopathic arthritis. J Rheumatol 2005;32(2):362–5.
66. Huppertz HI, Tschammler A, Horwiz AE, et al. Intraarticular corticosteroids for chronic arthritis in children: efficacy and effects on cartilage and growth. J Pediatr 1995;127:317.
67. Sherry DD, Stein LD, Reed AM, et al. Prevention of leg length discrepancy in young children with pauciarticular juvenile rheumatoid arthritis by treatment with intraarticular steroids. Arthritis Rheum 1999;42(11):2330–4.
68. Eyring EJ, Longert A, Bass J. Synovectomy in juvenile rheumatoid arthritis: indications and short term results. J Bone Joint Surg Am 1971;53:638.
69. Granberry WM, Brewer EJ. Results of synovectomy in children with rheumatoid arthritis. Clin Orthop 1974;101:120.
70. Panikkar KV, Taylor A, Kamath S. A comparison of open and arthroscopic ankle fusion. Foot Ankle Surg 2003;9(3):169–72.
71. Ansell M, Swann M. Management of chronic arthritis of children. J Bone Joint Surg 1983;65:536–43.
72. Witt JD, Swann M. Surgery in children. In: Isenberg DA, Maddison PJ, Woo P, et al, editors. Oxford textbook of Rheumatology. 3rd edition. Oxford (NY): Oxford University Press; 2004. p. 1223.
73. Drew SJ, Cohen B, Witt JD. Surgical management of adolescents with rheumatic disease. In: Isenberg DA, Miller JJ, editors. Adolescent Rheumatology. London: Martin Dunitz Ltd; 1999. p. 263.
74. Felix NA, Kitaoka HB. Ankle arthrodesis in patients with rheumatoid arthritis. Clin Orthop 1998;349:58–64.
75. Lachiewicz PF, Inglis AE, Ranawat CS, et al. Total ankle replacement in rheumatoid arthritis. J Bone Joint Surg 1984;66:340–3.
76. Mann JA, Chou LB, Ross SD. Foot and ankle surgery. In: Skinner HB, editor. Current diagnosis and treatment in orthopedics. 4th edition. New York: Lange Medical Books/McGraw-Hill Medical Pub; 2006. p. 504.
77. Crosby LA, Yee TC, Formanek TS, et al. Complications following arthroscopic ankle arthrodesis. Foot Ankle Int 1996;17(6):340–2.
78. Genovese MC. Treatment of rheumatoid arthritis. In: Firestein GS, Budd RC, Harris ED Jr, editors. Kelly's textbook of rheumatology. 8th edition. Philadelphia: W.B. Saunders; 2008. Chapter 67.
79. Wright DA. Juvenile idiopathic arthritis. In: Morrissy RT, Weinstein SL, editors, Lovell and Winter's pediatric orthopaedics, vol. 6. Philadelphia: Lippincott Williams & Wilkins; 2006. p. 405–37.
80. Karmazyn B, Bowyer SL, Schmidt KM, et al. US findings of metacarpophalangeal joints in children with idiopathic juvenile arthritis. Pediatr Radiol 2007;37:475–82.

Perioperative Management of the Patient with Rheumatoid Arthritis

Allen Mark Jacobs, DPM

KEYWORDS

- Complications • Medications • Perioperative management
- Rheumatoid arthritis

Rheumatoid arthritis is characterized by multiple joint involvement, and extraarticular manifestations are not infrequent. Systemic factors associated with rheumatoid arthritis may increase complication rates associated with surgery performed on the patient with this disorder. The results of surgery in a patient with rheumatoid arthritis are frequently less predictable in outcome than the same surgeries performed on a patient without rheumatoid arthritis. Prolonged recovery, and increased cost associated with the performance of surgery on the patient with rheumatoid arthritis is not uncommon.

The perioperative evaluation of the patient with rheumatoid arthritis involves the normal preoperative medical evaluation performed before any foot and ankle surgery, as well as an assessment of the level of disease activity, and evaluation of potential surgical implications of medications used to treat the patient with rheumatic disorders.

In some patients with rheumatoid arthritis, surgical decision making is based more on the overall status of the patient rather than clinical or radiographic assessment of the foot or ankle deformity. Case number 1 illustrates preoperative radiographs of a 73-year-old female with severe, rigid forefoot contractures, suffering from pain below several lesser metatarsal heads. She is frail, has severe deformities of the neck, shoulders, elbows and hands, lives alone, and cannot use crutches or gait-assistive devices. The digital and metacarpophalangeal joint deformities were not reducible, and pressure from her plantar lesions caused by prolapse metatarsal heads, rigid fused and contracted digits, and displaced fat pads, was relieved by osteotomy of the involved metatarsals elevating the entire rigid complex dorsally. This resulted in a complete resolution of the patient's preoperative symptoms. The surgical procedures were selected to allow the patient rapid recovery, immediate ambulation, without the need for any gait-assistive devices or immobilization.

6400 Clayton Road, Suite 402, St Louis, MO 63117, USA
E-mail address: drjacobs0902@sbcglobal.net

Clin Podiatr Med Surg 27 (2010) 235–242
doi:10.1016/j.cpm.2010.02.001
0891-8422/10/$ – see front matter © 2010 Published by Elsevier Inc.

podiatric.theclinics.com

Case number 2 involved a 40-year-old active female with severe deformities of her forefoot secondary to rheumatoid arthritis. She was felt to be a candidate for joint-sparing surgery primarily because of her young age and activity level. Entanercept was discontinued 1 month before surgery, and joint-sparing reduction of her deformities was performed with an excellent clinical outcome.

Case number 3 was an obese patient with rheumatoid arthritis, concurrent diabetes and multiple additional medical comorbidities. She suffered from a significant rearfoot valgus deformity that did not respond to bracing. Given her advanced age, diabetes, and obesity, she was not considered to be an ideal candidate for major rearfoot fusion. She was treated by a subtalar joint arthroereisis, which allowed immediate ambulation.

In each of these cases, the elected surgical intervention was determined as much by the patient's overall physical status, concurrent medical problems, and medications used, as any additional local factors.

Not infrequently, the patient with rheumatoid arthritis has thin atrophic skin and rigid long-standing contractures. Correction of deformities in such patients may be associated with neurologic or vascular insult because of long-standing contracture and sudden tensioning of these structures following surgical correction. The presence of thin atrophic skin with wasting of subcutaneous tissues may also prove problematic in providing coverage over fixation devices or implant devices. Poor wound healing may also be associated with such atrophic soft tissues.

Osteoporosis may be present as a result of disuse atrophy, the disease process, as well as the effects of medications used in the management of rheumatoid arthritis such as glucorticoids. In such patients, osteoporosis and osteopenia may result in poor fixation purchase and security, or implant instability within bone structures, necessitating the use of additional fixation, Kirschner wires, or Steinmann pins, autogenous or allogeneic bone grafting, or the use of orthobiologic substances.

Similarly, atrophic and weakened tendons may require orthobiologic supplementation for strength and to improve healing following reconstructive surgery.

Supplementation with calcium, vitamin D, or the use of substances such as calcitonin or bisphosphonate therapy may be required to prevent additional bone loss during the perioperative period. General nutritional therapy, such as vitamin D supplementation in the patient taking methotrexate, may also be required to achieve maximal healing.

GENERAL PATIENT CONSIDERATIONS

Many patients with rheumatoid arthritis are frail, and may not have the ability to use gait-assistive devices because of upper extremity, hip, or knee pathology. As a result, the academically ideal procedure may have to be modified to accommodate the general needs of the patient. The living environment of the patient and the presence or absence of support systems for daily activities while recovering from surgery should be assessed, and appropriate arrangements completed before embarking on significant surgical interventions in the patient with rheumatoid arthritis.

Cervical Spine Disease

Many patients with rheumatoid arthritis may have silent cervical spine disease. This may include atlantal-axial (C1–C2) subluxation which, if undetected, could result in significant tragic consequences following forceful manipulation of the head or neck in the perioperative period. When spinal anesthesia or general anesthesia is considered appropriate for a particular patient with rheumatoid arthritis, lateral radiographs of the cervical spine in full flexion and extension are recommended to assess the pre-odontoid space to evaluate the patient for the presence of atlantal axial subluxation. Anterior atlantoaxial subluxation is not rare in the patient with rheumatoid arthritis. As many as 80% of patients with rheumatoid arthritis may suffer from cervical spine disease. The greatest risk for cervical spine disease is present in the patient with neck symptoms, chronic erosive disease, a history of rheumatoid nodule formation, and elderly patients. Occipital pain or clicking of the neck with flexion and extension, and patient perception of anterior head subluxation are significant findings requiring evaluation of the cervical spine before surgical intervention.

MEDICATIONS

Medications used in the management of rheumatoid arthritis may include aspirin, nonsteroidal antiinflammatory medications, glucocorticoids, disease-modifying drugs (biologics). In addition, the patient may be taking a variety of over-the-counter medications or herbal medications. Failure to consider the medications that a patient is using for the treatment of rheumatoid arthritis, and failure to make appropriate modifications in such medications when necessary, may increase the risk for operative complications. Case 4 illustrates a significant hematoma and eventual ischemia that occurred in the great toe of a patient with rheumatoid arthritis and diabetes who was taking aspirin that was not discontinued before surgical intervention.

Aspirin and Antiinflammatory Medications

Aspirin and antiinflammatory medications, including Cox-2 selective medications, act by inhibiting the synthesis of prostaglandins. Tissue injury results in the cleavage of arachadonic acid from cell walls by the activity of phospholipase A2, a cleaving enzyme. The activity of phospholipase A2 is inhibited by the administration of glucocorticoids. Once formed, arachadonic acid is acted on by local isomerases to form various prostaglandins that are tissue specific. For example, antiinflammatory medications block the synthesis of thromboxane A2 in platelets, thereby interfering with platelet aggregation and clot formation, increasing the risk of bleeding. The result of failing to discontinue aspirin or antiinflammatory medications before surgery may be associated with increased risk of bleeding, hematoma, and hematoma-associated complications.

In general, aspirin should be discontinued 10 days before surgery because it irreversibly binds thromboxane A2. As a result, platelets will not function properly leading to increased risk of postoperative hemorrhage and hematoma. Prompt re-initiation of aspirin therapy is generally recommended when the risk of hemorrhage following surgery is diminished. There is a higher frequency of excessive operative hemorrhage when aspirin is used in combination with other antiplatelet medications, in a patient with preexisting hepatic or renal disease, or patients with known unknown preexisting coagulation disorders.

Nonselective antiinflammatory medications generally reversibly inhibit thromboxane A2. As a general rule, nonselective antiinflammatory medications should be discontinued 5 half-lives before surgery. Examples are ibuprofen, which should be discontinued 1 or 2 days before surgery, naproxen which should be discontinued 3 days before surgery, sulindac 4 days before surgery, nabumetone 5 days before surgery, piroxicam and oxaprozin 10 days before surgical intervention.

Cox-2 should be similarly treated, although selective Cox-2 inhibitors do not seem to affect platelets as greatly as nonselective antiinflammatories and may not need to be discontinued before some foot or ankle surgical interventions.[1]

When concerns exist about the effects of these medications relative to operative bleeding, preoperative bleeding times may be considered but the results of such studies have been generally shown not to be predictive of operative healing time. In general, antiinflammatory medications are considered to be associated with increased risk of operative hemorrhage.[2–5]

Glucocorticoids

It is vital to maintain glucocorticoid therapy during the entire perioperative period. Discontinuation of even low doses of glucocorticoids may result in a significant flare of disease activity with profound clinical consequences. In addition, abrupt withdrawal of corticosteroid therapy in the perioperative period may result in acute adrenocortical crisis.

Generally, 20 to 30 mg of glucocorticoids are synthesized daily by the adrenal cortex in response to stimulation by adrenocorticotropic hormone. Adrenocorticotropic hormone is released by the anterior pituitary gland in response to corticotrophin-releasing hormone from the hypothalamus, which itself is released in response to serum cortical levels. Prolonged exogenous corticosteroid exposure results in suppression of the ability of the adrenal cortex to intrinsically produce group corticoids through physiologic and true anatomic atrophy. Glucorticoids are required to respond to stress. In the absence of the ability of the adrenal cortex to produce glucocorticoids, the absent glucorticoid response to stress may result in significant mortality and morbidity. Elevated levels of the corticoids are necessary at the time of incision, during surgery in general, during the reversal of anesthesia, during extirpation, and during the postoperative period.

In the patient who has been taking 5 mg per day or less of corticosteroids, and in whom podiatric surgery is less than 1 hour, and is to be performed under local anesthesia, no glucocorticoid supplementation is required.[6]

Generally, when glucocorticoid therapy supplementation is required, lower doses and shorter duration of glucocorticoid supplementation is recommended than those that have been traditionally taught in textbooks. For most podiatric surgical procedures, 25 mg of hydrocortisone or 5 mg of methylprednisolone administered intravenously before surgery likely provides sufficient prophylaxis. For moderately stressful procedures such as major rearfoot fusion, or ankle implant arthroplasty, 50 to 75 mg of hydrocortisone, or 10 to 15 mg of methyl prednisolone may be administered intravenously before surgery, with the dose rapidly tapered over the ensuing 24 to 48 hours.[7]

Methotrexate

The effects of methotrexate on surgery performed in the patient with rheumatoid arthritis remains controversial. Retrospective studies on the use of methotrexate in the perioperative period have demonstrated increased incidence of infection and wound-healing complications, and no effect of methotrexate has been demonstrated during the perioperative period. In general, it is now considered that methotrexate is not associated with increased risk of infection or increased risk of poor wound healing. Methotrexate may be continued through the perioperative period in most patients. It should be withheld in elderly patients, frail patients, or those with renal insufficiency. If concern exists in a particular patient regarding wound healing or infectious complications, consideration may be given to the discontinuation of methotrexate 4 weeks before surgery.[8–11]

Penicillamine

Penicillamine may be associated with increased risk of delayed wound healing. In patients taking penicillamine, consideration should be given to delaying removal of sutures, and perhaps more vigorous detailed suture support during wound closure.

Tumor Necrosis Factor-α-, β Inhibitors and Biologics

Tumor necrosis factor inhibitors have become increasingly used for the management of rheumatoid arthritis and other disorders. These agents suppress the inflammatory response and are therefore helpful in diminishing destruction secondary to rheumatoid arthritis. However, they also reduced normal inflammation required for wound healing, and as a result may be associated with increased risk of infectious complications or wound-healing complications. Although somewhat controversial, it is generally considered appropriate to discontinue tumor necrosis factor inhibitors before surgery and to continue discontinuation of these agents until healing has been accomplished. It is also felt that these agents should not be reinstituted while there are any exposed Kirschner wires, external fixation devices, or any open wound or infectious process in the perioperative period.

Commonly employed biologics for the treatment of rheumatoid arthritis include entanercept (Enbrel) and infliximab (Remicade), adalimumab (Humira), abatacept (Orencia).

Increased incidence of infectious complications in patients taking tumor necrosis factor inhibitors has been reported, however, some investigators have suggested that the discontinuation of tumor necrosis factor inhibitors is not required or necessary in the perioperative period for foot and ankle surgery in a patient with rheumatoid arthritis.[12–15]

Interleukin-1 inhibitors include anakindra (Kineret) and atlizumab (Actmera) which should also be discontinued before surgical intervention because of interference with the inflammatory process and subsequent potential sequela.

Other agents used to treat rheumatoid arthritis include hydroxychloroquine, which may be continued throughout the perioperative period. Sulfasalazine should be discontinued about 4 or 5 days before surgery, as should azathioprine. Leflunamide and cyclophosphamide should be discontinued 1 or 2 weeks before surgical intervention.

LABORATORY STUDIES

Laboratory abnormalities are not uncommon in a patient with rheumatoid arthritis and may create difficulties in the interpretation of laboratory studies following surgery when complications are being evaluated. Common laboratory abnormalities in the patient with rheumatoid arthritis include leukocytosis associated with the disease, thrombocytosis, and normochromic anemia. An increase in the erythrocyte sedimentation rate or C reactive protein level may be associated with the disease process making the interpretation of such studies more difficult when problems such as infection are being considered.

DEEP VEIN THROMBOPHLEBITIS

Many patients undergoing reconstructive surgery of the foot and ankle for rheumatoid arthritis are immobilized for prolonged periods of time as a consequence of such surgery. In addition, patients with significant deformity may suffer from generalized immobility because of the nature of their disease with superimposed postoperative immobility. In those patients felt to be at increased risk for thrombosis, consideration should be given to prophylactic therapy in an effort to reduce the incidence of deep vein thrombosis. Such measures may range from 2 aspirin daily, administration of warfarin (Coumadin), or the use of a traditional agents such as dalteparin (Fragmin) or enoxaparin (Lovenox).

OPERATIVE COMPLICATIONS

Several studies have suggested that the patient with rheumatoid arthritis undergoing elective surgery of the foot and ankle is at risk for increased rate of complications, including infection and poor wound healing.

Overall, the largest study of complications following surgery on the patient with rheumatoid arthritis undergoing foot and ankle surgery reports a complication rate of 32%.[16] Wound-healing complications represented most of such problems. No association with age, duration of disease, or the use of any particular medication has been firmly established. In the patient with rheumatoid arthritis, a 14% infection rate has been reported following pan metatarsal head resection,[17] and a 12% infection rate has been reported following tibialtalocalcaneal fusion.[18]

As a general rule, prophylaxis should be administered before surgery on the patient with rheumatoid arthritis. Such prophylaxis should be directed at staphylococcal and streptococcal organisms.

Delayed Union and Nonunion

Although the patient with rheumatoid arthritis suffers from atrophic tissues, and the effects of medications such as corticoids on bone and joint structures, a significant risk for delayed union or nonunion following osteotomy or arthrodesis procedures has not been reported in patient with rheumatoid arthritis.

Vascular Complications

Rheumatoid arthritis may be associated with Raynaud phenomena, vasculitis, or vasospasm. When present, use of cold therapy following surgery should be interdicted. Because many of the deformities in the rheumatoid forefoot are extensive, and have been present for many years, sudden reduction of these deformities may result in traction or tension on soft tissues such as vascular structures resulting in ischemia. When significant deformities are reduced at the time of surgery, care must be taken to monitor such patients for the presence of acute vascular compromise and to provide appropriate interdiction to avoid serious complications such as gangrene. Vasculitis, in particular, is more common in male patients, those with high titer rheumatoid factor, patients with significant joint erosive disease, and in those patients with rheumatoid nodules or other extraarticular manifestations.

Neurologic Complications

The patient with rheumatoid arthritis may suffer from peripheral neuropathy secondary to the disease process, entrapment neuropathy such as tarsal tunnel syndrome, or the neuropathic effects of medication used to treat the disease process. The presence of such neurologic sequelae of the rheumatoid process should be recognized before surgery and considered as a possible cause of patient discomfort. Interdigital neuroma formation has been reported as occurring with increased frequency in a patient with rheumatoid arthritis, in addition to which soft tissue pathology such as rheumatoid nodules or synovitis adjacent to articular structures may result in secondary nerve compression syndromes with associated neurologic manifestations.

Tendon Pathology

Inflammatory disorders of tendons, as well as partial or total rupture of tendon structures may occur in association with rheumatoid arthritis or result secondarily from corticosteroid injections or systemic corticoid therapy. Consideration should be given to the evaluation of tendon pathology with magnetic resonance imaging (MRI) or diagnostic ultrasound studies before surgical intervention when appropriate (eg, patients in whom tendon transfer or lengthening is considered).

Soft Tissue Pathology

A variety of soft tissue pathologic conditions such as synovitis of joint structures, tenosynovitis, and bursitis occur with increased frequency in a patient with rheumatoid arthritis. When suspected, soft tissue pathology may be evaluated initially by standard radiographs supplemented by diagnostic ultrasonography or MRI studies.

SUMMARY

Familiarity with the systemic manifestations of rheumatoid arthritis as well as familiarity with drug therapy used for the management of rheumatoid arthritis may be helpful in the avoidance of some postoperative complications. Drug effects on soft tissues and bone may complicate reduction, stabilization, and fixation of deformities. Evaluation of the patient with rheumatoid arthritis for extraarticular disease may also explain symptomatology, and reduce the incidence of complications by unrecognized contributions of soft tissue pathology of osseous and articular disorders.

REFERENCES

1. Kelley JT, Conn DL. Perioperative management of the rheumatic disease patient. Bull Rheum Dis 2002;51(6):I–7.
2. Lind SE. The bleeding time does not predict surgical bleeding. Blood 1991;77: 2547.
3. Gerwirtz AS, Miller ML, Keys TF. The clinical usefulness of the preoperative bleeding time. Arch Pathol Lab Med 1996;120:353–6.
4. Connelly CS, Panush RS. Should nonsteroidal anti-inflammatory drugs be stopped before elective surgery? Arch Intern Med 1991;151:1963–6.
5. Robinson CM, Christie J, Malcolm-Smith N. Nonsteroidal antiinflammatory drugs, perioperative blood loss, and transfusion requirements in elective hip arthroplasty. J Arthroplasty 1993;8:607–10.
6. Coursin DB, Wood KE. Corticosteroid supplementation for adrenal insufficiency. JAMA 2002;287:236.
7. Lamberts SW, Bruining HA, de Jong FH. Corticosteroid therapy in severe illness. N Engl J Med 1997;337:1285–92.
8. Perhala RS, Wilke WS, Clough JD, et al. Local infectious complications following knee joint replacement in rheumatoid arthritis patients treated with methotrexate versus those not treated with methotrexate. Arthritis Rheum 1991;34:146.
9. Kasdan ML, June L. Postoperative results of rheumatoid arthritis patients on methotrexate at the time of reconstructive surgery of the hand. Orthopedics 1993;16:1233–5.
10. Grennan DM, Gray J, Loudon J, et al. Methotrexate and early postoperative complications in patients with rheumatoid arthritis undergoing elective orthopaedic surgery. Ann Rheum Dis 2001;60:214–7.
11. Bibbo C. Wound healing complications and infection following surgery for rheumatoid arthritis. Foot Ankle Clin 2007;12(3):509–24.
12. Lee RH, Efron DT, Tantry U, et al. Inhibition of tumor necrosis factor-alpha attenuates wound breaking strength in rats. Wound Repair Regen 2000;8:547–53.
13. Dixon W, Watson K, Lunt M, et al. Serious infection rates, including site-specific and bacterial intracellular infection rates, in rheumatoid arthritis patients treated

with anti-TNFαtherapy: results from the British Society for Rheumatology Biologies Register (BSRBR). Arthritis Rheum 2006;54:2368–76.

14. Listing J, Strangfeld A, Kary S, et al. Infections in patients with rheumatoid arthritis treated with biologic agents. Arthritis Rheum 2005;52(I I):3403–12.

15. Crawford M, Curtis JR. Tumor necrosis factor inhibitors and infection complications. Curr Rheumatol Rep 2008;10:383–9.

16. Bibbo C, Anderson RB, Davis WH. Injury characteristics and the clinical outcome of subtalar dislocations: a clinical and radiographic analysis of 25 cases. Foot Ankle Int 2003;24(2):158–63.

17. Reize P, Ina Leichtle C, Leichtle UG, et al. Long-term results after metatarsal head resection in the treatment of rheumatoid arthritis. Foot Ankle Int 2006;27(8): 586–90.

18. Anderson T, Linder L, Rydholm U, et al. Tibio-talocalcaneal arthrodesis as a primary procedure using a retrograde intramedullary nail: a retrospective study of 26 patients with rheumatoid arthritis. Acta Orthop 2005;76:580–7.

The Surgical Reconstruction of the Rheumatoid Forefoot

Alfonso Anthony Haro, III, DPM[a],*, Lacey F. Moore, MD[b],
Karen Schorn, MD[c], Lawrence A. DiDomenico, DPM[d]

KEYWORDS

- Rheumatoid arthritis • Rheumatoid foot • Forefoot surgery
- Forefoot deformity • Forefoot reconstruction

Rheumatoid arthritis (RA) is reported to affect 0.5% to 1% of the population.[1–7] This disease begins in the foot approximately 20% of the time,[8,9] and results in work disability in greater than 50% of patients[1–3] and foot deformity in approximately 100% of patients within 10 years of the onset of the disease.[4,10–13] The forefoot is more often affected than the rearfoot,[4,8,9] with 70% to 80% of the metatarsophalangeal (MTP) joints being involved early in the disease process,[14,15] resulting in the development of deformities in 90% of adults with chronic RA.[16,17] RA is an autoimmune disorder that presents in females more often than in males and may affect any age to include infants, but is primarily noted in the fourth and the fifth decades and provides no regional or ethnic preference.[18] Although genetic and environmental causes have been proposed, the definitive cause of immunologic susceptibility, as well as viral and bacterial infectious processes that may cause RA, have not been identified.[1,18]

PURPOSE

This article discusses reconstructive forefoot surgery for RA via soft-tissue procedures, joint-destructive procedures, and joint-sparing procedures, and highlights the combined approaches to reconstruction via forefoot joint-sparing techniques using soft-tissue rebalancing in conjunction with first ray forefoot joint-sparing procedures

[a] Ankle and Foot Surgical and Podiatry Clinic, 200 Westgate Drive, Suite A, West End, NC 27376, USA
[b] Pinehurst Radiology, 30 Memorial Drive, Pinehurst, NC 28374, USA
[c] Pinehurst Rheumatology Clinic, 681 South Bennett Street, Southern Pines, NC 28387, USA
[d] Ankle and Foot and Care Centers, Northside Medical Center Forum Health, 500 Gypsy Lane, Youngstown, OH 44501, USA
* Corresponding author.
E-mail address: alfonsoaharoiii@aol.com

Clin Podiatr Med Surg 27 (2010) 243–259
doi:10.1016/j.cpm.2009.12.007
0891-8422/10/$ – see front matter © 2010 Elsevier Inc. All rights reserved.

podiatric.theclinics.com

and midfoot joint-destructive procedures. This article also includes a discussion of the radiographic and magnetic resonance imaging (MRI) findings associated with RA and a discussion of perioperative care for the RA patient undergoing forefoot surgery.

CLINICAL PRESENTATION AND DIAGNOSIS

The various pathologies of RA of the forefoot that may be encountered include rheumatoid nodules; synovitis; pannus; capsulitis; bursitis; edema; metatarsalgia; fat pad migration and atrophy; calluses; ulceration; infection; hallux abducto valgus; hammertoe, claw toe, or mallet toe deformities; MTP joint soft tissue, cartilage, and bone erosion; and joint contractures, subluxations, or dislocations. The severity of the pathology may range from mild swelling and early joint pain with no or limited deformity to more pronounced swelling and severe joint pain, or absence of joint pain with mild to severe joint deformity with or without joint destruction. Pathologies of the lower extremity that may be found in the rheumatoid patient include osteoporosis, vasculitis and atherosclerosis, and cervical spine disease, as well as neuropathy that is secondary to entrapment, vasculitis, or drug toxicity.[18]

No single diagnostic test is provided to definitively diagnose RA. The American Rheumatism Association has provided 7 criteria and the corresponding definitions of each criterion for the classification of RA, and these may be used to assist in making the diagnosis. To be classified as having RA a person must exhibit 4 of the 7 qualifying criteria that include morning stiffness, arthritis of 3 or more joint areas, arthritis of hand joints, symmetric arthritis, rheumatoid nodules, and serum rheumatoid factor. Of these criteria the first 4 must be present for a minimum of 6 weeks.[1,19,20] Patients displaying 2 of the satisfying criteria are not excluded from the diagnosis of RA.[1] Also of note, arthritis of the hand joints is included as one of the first 4 qualifying criteria that is required to be present for at least 6 weeks, whereas arthritis of the foot joints is not specifically required despite the fact that foot has been reported to be the first affected site in up to 19% of patients, with 21% of patients developing pedal pathology within the first year of the disease process.[4]

IMAGING FINDINGS OF RA IN THE FOREFOOT

RA involves the feet in up to 90% of patients, usually just lagging behind the hands in terms of frequency of involvement. Radiographic features of the involvement of the forefoot in RA are nonspecific; however, the constellation of findings together with clinical suspicion will often support the diagnosis. Early in the disease process, radiographs show periarticular osteopenia about the MTP joints. This finding reflects that synovitis and associated hyperemia occur about the joint, thus causing a washout of bone mineralization. Soft-tissue swelling about the MTP joints may also be appreciated. As the disease process progresses, marginal erosions become detectable. These erosions are first seen at the bare areas of the metatarsal heads, with the lateral aspect of the fifth metatarsal head usually being the first to be involved. **Fig. 1** shows periarticular osteopenia with small marginal erosions involving the fifth metatarsal head. Progressive erosive changes will usually be more extensive along the medial metatarsal heads as compared with the lateral aspects. No new bone production is seen about the erosive change. More progressive involvement of the forefoot will show a uniform and symmetric loss of the MTP joint space. As the MTP joint cartilage is destroyed, lateral subluxation of the proximal phalanges will be apparent. Hallux valgus and proximal interphalangeal joint dorsiflexion deformities may also be seen late in the disease process. Very late changes include severe periarticular erosions involving the MTP joints with associated lateral subluxations. Findings are symmetric

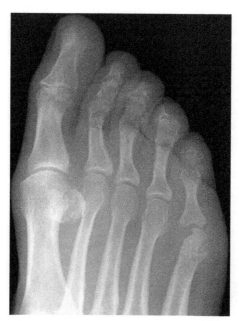

Fig. 1. Radiograph showing periarticular osteopenia with small marginal erosions involving the fifth metatarsal head.

with the contralateral forefoot. **Fig. 2** shows the late changes of RA in the forefoot, with extensive loss of MTP joint space of the second through fifth digits and marked erosive change about these joints.[21] MRI is being increasingly used to detect the first manifestations of RA in the forefoot, and it shows periarticular bone marrow edema and synovitis that affect the MTP joint before appreciable periarticular osteopenia or small marginal erosions are detectable on radiographs. Tenosynovitis is often associated and can easily be detected with MRI. Some researchers have advocated MRI as the gold standard for the detection and characterization of RA affecting the joints.[18] Although MRI is clearly more sensitive than radiographs, it is more costly and not as readily available. MRI certainly has an important role in problem solving.

In summary, radiographic manifestations of early RA in the forefoot include MTP joint periarticular osteopenia with associated small marginal erosions about the metatarsal heads, first along the lateral fifth metatarsal head. As the disease progresses, erosions become more extensive and lateral subluxation of the proximal phalanges develop. Uniform MTP joint space narrowing is evident. Findings are seen to be symmetric with the contralateral foot. Findings can usually be distinguished from psoriatic and reactive arthritis, as bone mineral density is preserved in psoriasis and there is bone production about the areas of erosive change in psoriasis and reactive arthritis. These arthropathies are also bilaterally asymmetric. Collagen vascular diseases are not usually a diagnostic dilemma, as these do not show erosive change or loss of joint space.

PRE- AND POSTOPERATIVE CONSIDERATIONS FOR THE MEDICAL MANAGEMENT OF THE PATIENT WITH PODIATRIC RA

RA is a common inflammatory joint disease that affects approximately 1% of the population and 3% of the population older than 65 years.[22] Irreversible structural damage

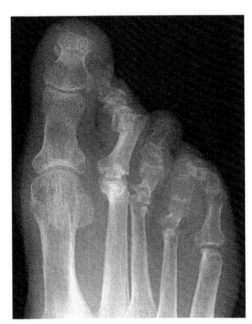

Fig. 2. Late changes of RA in the forefoot with extensive loss of MTP joint space of the second through fifth digits and marked erosive change about these joints. (*Data from* Brower AC. Arthritis in black and white. Philadelphia: WB Saunders; 1988.)

arising from synovitis frequently requires surgical intervention. The need for surgical intervention tends to occur later in the disease. Patients with RA have elective surgery for 2 primary reasons, namely to relieve pain and to improve functional status.

Patients with RA have a higher risk of postsurgical complications, including wound healing, because of their underlying systemic disease, immunosuppressive medications, malnutrition, and often severe deformities that need corrective surgery. Nonunion occurs in rheumatoid patients at a higher rate than the general population. This nonunion is thought to be caused by the same factors that cause postsurgical complications.[23,24]

Preoperative evaluation and medical management should focus on optimizing the patient's medical condition to reduce the risk of complications. Patients should be evaluated for skin ulcerations, vasculitis, carious teeth, periodontal disease, urinary tract infection, or prostatism, because these problems can increase the risk of postoperative infections.[25]

Cervical spine involvement merits careful attention in RA patients no matter what type of surgery is planned. Thirty to forty percent of patients with RA have cervical spine involvement, which is often asymptomatic.[26] An unstable cervical spine from atlantoaxial or subaxial subluxation places the patient at an increased risk for neurologic complications, especially with endotracheal intubation. Care should be taken during spinal anesthesia not to cause unnecessary prolonged flexion of the cervical spine. It is recommended that cervical radiography in lateral flexion and extension be conducted before surgery.[27]

Preoperative evaluation recommendations for patients with RA include electrocardiography, prothrombin time, partial thromboplastin time, complete blood count with platelets, electrolytes, creatinine, liver function tests, chest radiograph, cervical spine radiograph, and skin evaluation to look for ulcerations, nodules, skin break-down, or vasculitis. Lung involvement is common in RA and may not be apparent because of the patient's functional limitations. The rheumatoid patient is at an increased risk of developing pulmonary problems perioperatively if interstitial fibrosis is present; this affects gas exchange by decreasing the diffusion capacity.[28]

Blood loss is an inevitable consequence of surgery, and a hemoglobin level less than 13 predicts a 2-fold increase in the need for a transfusion in most orthopedic procedures.

Steroids should be maintained at the lowest possible dose before surgery. Nonsteroidal anti-inflammatory drugs (NSAIDs) should be discontinued 5 or more days before the procedure. Aspirin needs to be held for 1 week before the procedure. NSAIDs inhibit thromboxane A_2 synthesis and can prolong bleeding time. Stress dose of the steroid hydrocortisone (100 mg) should be given intravenously (IV) before surgery. If the procedure is prolonged then hydrocortisone IV (100 mg) should be given intraoperatively. Hydrocortisone IV (100 mg) should be continued at an interval of 8 hours for 24 hours. If the patient is not allowed to take in food orally, then hydrocortisone (IV) (50 mg) should be given every 8 hours for 24 hours; however, if he can take food through the mouth, the usual oral dose of prednisone can be resumed. Recent studies suggest that patients who discontinued methotrexate before surgery had more postoperative infections and complications than patients who continued methotrexate.[29,30] Use of disease-modifying antirheumatic drugs (DMARDs), such as penicillamine, cyclosporine, and antimalarials, were associated with an increased risk of postoperative infections Agents that can cause leukopenia, namely cyclophosphamide (Cytoxan), azathioprine (Imuran), and sulfasalazine (Azulfidine), should be discontinued a few days preoperatively. At present there are no data on the use of leflunomide in the perioperative period, but it is currently recommended to hold the drug 2 weeks prior to elective surgery and resume its use when the patient is able to take oral medication.[31] The biologic DMARDs such as tumor necrosis factor (TNF) inhibitors and interleukin (IL)-1 have a significant impact on the treatment of RA. Proinflammatory cytokines, IL-1, and TNF-α play a central role in the pathophysiology of RA. These biologic therapies have a rapid onset and have been shown to prevent structural damage in RA. However, their main side effect is an increased risk of infection. It is recommended that these drugs should be administered for 1 dosing interval only, that is, etanercept for 1 week, adalimumab for 2 to 4 weeks, and infliximab for 6 to 8 weeks. Elective surgery is not advised when the drugs are at peak levels in the therapy. These TNFs can be reinstated 2 weeks after surgery as long as the wound is clean and healing well.

Rehabilitation is recommended after most surgeries, and follow-up radiographs are screened to document healing.

Rheumatoid flares that occur during the peri- or postoperative period can be managed with corticosteroids.

SURGICAL INTERVENTION

If conservative pressure reducing and offloading modalities, such as callous debridement, padding, accommodative or custom shoes, and custom orthotics, as well as pharmacologic management fail to alleviate symptomatic RA forefoot pathology, surgical intervention is indicated with the goal of reducing pain and recreation of a plantar grade foot that may be fitted with a shoe. Care must be taken to adequately assess the patient's vascular status, because vasculitis may be present and should be accounted for when selecting a surgical procedure that balances the desired deformity correction and wound-healing potential.

Removal of Soft Tissue Nodules or Masses

The literature indicates that 20% to 32% of patients with RA present with rheumatoid nodules, which are usually not painful.[18,32] Rheumatoid nodules result from a vasculitic process and have been reported to be a sign of an advanced stage of RA.[33–35] A study by Bibbo and colleagues[33] found that rheumatoid nodules were present in 43% of 104 patients. They reported that there was no statistically significant difference in the frequency of occurrence of rheumatoid nodules between groups of patients with postoperative complications and groups of patients without postoperative complications, and that there were fewer postoperative complications in the group of patients who had had rheumatoid nodules. Rheumatoid nodules located in weight-bearing regions may be symptomatic and predispose one to pain, ulceration, and infection. **Fig. 3** displays the rheumatoid nodules in plantar forefoot. Surgical removal of rheumatoid nodules or masses is performed by excising the identified soft-tissue nodule via the most direct approach, with the goal of producing the least soft-tissue damage and with consideration given to the surrounding anatomic structures, weight-bearing verses nonweight-bearing surfaces, relaxed skin tension lines, and the potential need for additional incision placement and reconstructive forefoot surgery. Postoperative care must be given to protect incisions from excessive tension, shear, and friction to provide maximum opportunity for skin healing and acceptable scar formation, especially in cases where a plantar approach is used. Three weeks of nonweight bearing on plantar incisions is recommended to assist in avoiding hypertrophic and painful scar formation. **Fig. 4** displays the plantar forefoot scar post resection of the rheumatoid nodules that had been identified previously.

Classic incision approaches of interest in rheumatoid forefoot surgery include Hoffman's (1912) distal transverse plantar incision; Larmon's (1951) 3 dorsal longitudinal incisions; Fowler's (1959) distal transverse dorsal incision with first and fifth ray longitudinal extensions and a plantar skin ellipse; Clayton's (1960) distal transverse dorsal incision; and Kates' (1967) curved plantar incision with a plantar ellipse.[20] The surgical authors prefer the use of 2 dorsal foot incisions of which 1 dorsal forefoot incision is modeled after a single incision introduced by Hibbs in 1919 for the treatment of clawfoot.[36,37] The dorsal modified Hibbs incision extends from the distal medial second metatarsal head region to proximal lateral region; spanning the second, third, fourth, and fifth metatarsals and providing access to the corresponding MTP joints and digital

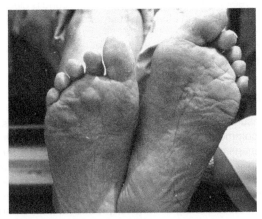

Fig. 3. Rheumatoid nodules in a patient with plantar forefoot.

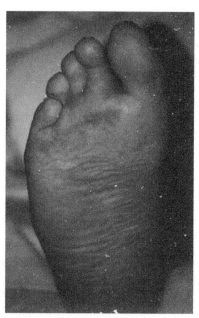

Fig. 4. The plantar forefoot scar post resection of the previously identified rheumatoid nodules.

extensor tendons for soft-tissue rebalancing. It is combined with a second dorsal medial longitudinal first ray incision, which provides access to the joints of the medial column and first MTP joint as needed for stabilization. **Fig. 5** displays a healed modified Hibbs incision on the right foot and a healed dorsal medial longitudinal first ray incision on the left foot.

Correction of Digital Pathology

Correction of hammertoe, claw toe, and mallet toe may be achieved via independent procedures or by combinations of procedures, such as an arthroplasty,

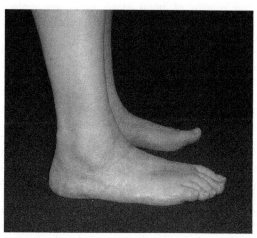

Fig. 5. Healed modified Hibbs incision on the right foot and a healed dorsal medial longitudinal first ray incision on the left foot.

arthrodesis, osteoclasis, flexor digitorum tenotomy, flexor digitorum longus tendon transfer, flexor hallucis longus tendon transfer or capsulotomy of the distal interphalangeal joint, proximal interphalangeal joint, and hallux interphalangeal joints. The approach to hammertoe correction varies and is based on surgeon's preference, global surgical planning, and patient suitability. The planned approach to digital correction should take into account the desired goal, surgeon's experience, the digital pathology that is presented, the patient's vascular status, the patient's health, as well as the operative time that is required if additional surgical reconstructive procedures need to be performed. The surgical approach may be modified to address the presentation of reducible, semireducible, or fixed nonreducible hammertoes with or without additional MTP pathology, hallux abducto valgus, and first ray stability.

The digital joint-destructive procedures include arthroplasty, implant arthroplasty, and arthrodesis. Although the surgical authors prefer joint-sparing procedures, proximal interphalangeal joint arthroplasty when required is the digital joint-destructive procedure of choice in the RA population. Digital arthroplasty usually involves removal of the head of the proximal phalanx and less often the head of the distal phalanx via a dorsal curvilinear or longitudinal incision on the second, third, fourth, and/or fifth digits, followed by 3 to 4 weeks of temporary Kirschner fixation with either a 0.045-in or 0.062-in wire. Digital implant arthroplasty may be performed; however, it is rarely recommended by the surgical authors. Arthrodesis of the digits typically involves removal of the cartilaginous surfaces and bone from the adjacent sides of the proximal interphalangeal joint, followed by bony realignment and apposition of the surface of the base of the intermediate phalanx and remaining distal aspect of the proximal phalanx. Arthrodesis in the RA population may be accomplished via various techniques and is often performed via end-to-end bony apposition rather than peg and hole bony apposition, then followed by Kirschner wire fixation. Additional methods of digital fixation include the use of specialized digital screws placed from distal to proximal spanning the distal, intermediate, and proximal phalanx, or the use of specialized locking intramedullary digital implants placed within the proximal shaft of the intermediate phalanx and the distal shaft of the proximal phalanx. With the digital arthrodesis approach the surgical authors' preference is end-to-end arthrodesis with Kirschner wire fixation in the RA population, because of the quality of bone stock often encountered and the high frequency of Kirschner wire use for temporary fixation of proximal MTP joint pathology that is often corrected at the same surgical setting. **Fig. 6** displays the reduced digital and MTP pathology with Kirschner wire fixation in place. Clayton presented the forefoot resection arthroplasty to the American Rheumatism Association in 1958, and the technique was later printed in *Clinical Orthopaedics and Related Research* in 1960. The Clayton procedure included MTP joint resections and digital arthroplasties in which the base of the proximal phalanx of the digits 1, 2, 3, 4, and 5 were resected, in conjunction with the resection of metatarsal heads 1, 2, 3, 4, and 5.[38,39] Complications, such as recurring hallux abducto valgus, development of floppy toes, and cockup digital deformities are noted to have led to the transition from simple forefoot resection procedures to reconstructive surgery during the latter portion of the 1970s.[39] The surgical authors guard against the use of the original Clayton procedure because of its joint-destructive nature and the resulting destabilization of the MTP joints. On the contrary, they favor forefoot joint-sparing reconstructive techniques that use the release of joint contractures and tendon rebalancing techniques for the lesser digits and lesser MTP joints, combined with first ray stabilizing procedures.

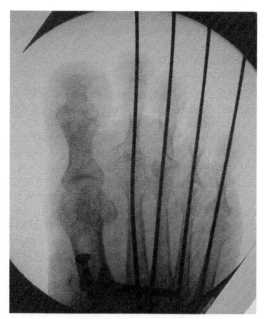

Fig. 6. The reduced digital and MTP pathology with Kirschner wire fixation in place.

Joint-Sparing Digital Procedures

Joint-sparing hammertoe correction is based on soft-tissue rebalancing and may be accomplished by performing open, percutaneous, or closed procedures that are aimed at releasing and reducing capsular and tendon contractures as well as reducing deforming soft-tissue influences by balancing tendon forces. Percutaneous plantar digital tenotomies, capsulotomies, and Kirschner wire fixation are often useful in reducing distal interphalangeal joint contractures and proximal interphalangeal joint contractures, and have been found to be useful in reducing operative time and soft-tissue trauma when combined with open MTP joint and proximal first ray procedures. Open distal interphalangeal joint and proximal interphalangeal joint capsulotomies, flexor digitorum longus tendon transfers, and percutaneous or open temporary Kirschner wire fixation are additional joint preserving approaches that are used to reduce hammertoes and claw toes. Flexor digitorum longus tendon transfers may be accomplished via various techniques such as a splint medial and lateral tendon transfer, complete medial or complete lateral tendon transfer, or dorsal tendon transfer through a bone tunnel. Of the 3 transfer options noted the surgical authors prefer an intact flexor digitorum longus tendon transfer, with the tendon being transferred to the proximal base of the proximal phalanx opposite the side of the primary deforming force. Therefore, if the deforming force is primarily plantar or plantarlateral, the flexor digitorum longus tendon is transferred to the proximal medial base of the proximal phalanx and the opposite is done if the deforming force is primarily plantarmedial. When harvesting the flexor digitorum longus for transfer the incision is performed on the plantar medial or lateral aspect of the digit according to the planned side of transfer, and is released from the distal phalanx distal to the distal interphalangeal joint, then transferred and reapproximated to the appropriate dorsal side of the proximal phalanx proximal to the proximal interphalangeal joint. After performing the flexor digitorum longus transfer a distal interphalangeal joint and proximal interphalangeal joint plantar capsulotomy is performed, and the digit is temporarily fixated in a rectus position by a Kirschner wire before coapting the tendon to the new insertion location.

CORRECTION OF MTP JOINT PATHOLOGY
MTP Joint-Destructive Procedures

Resection of the metatarsals was initially described by Hoffman[40] in 1912 whereby the metatarsal heads 1, 2, 3, 4, and 5 are transected and removed.[41] As previously mentioned, Clayton expanded on the metatarsal head resections by removing the bases of the adjacent proximal phalanxes.[38] Additional modifications to the original Hoffman procedure allow for combination resection of the metatarsal heads 2, 3, 4, and 5 with various first ray procedures to include resection of the base of the proximal phalanx of the hallux, first MTP joint implant arthroplasty, and first MTP joint arthrodesis. **Fig. 7** displays 5 resected metatarsal heads along with the base of the proximal phalanx of the hallux. The Keller resection arthroplasty and the first MTP joint implant arthroplasty are joint-destructive options. However, the surgical authors prefer the first MTP joint arthrodesis, which if successfully accomplished provides an increased medial column stability, alleviates approximately 50% hallux abducto valgus recurrence rate noted with arthroplasty procedures, and allows the first ray to share a greater load of weight-bearing forces.[4,17] The key to forefoot reconstruction in the rheumatoid patient is the achievement of a stable realigned first ray.[8,17] MTP joint preparation may be completed by mechanical debridement of cartilage with hand instrumentation, such as curettes, rongeurs, osteotomes, and rasps, or with power instrumentation such as sagittal saw resection, conical reaming devices, and burrs. Various fixation techniques may be used for the first MTP joint arthrodesis including crossed Kirschner wire fixation, Steinmann pin fixation, crossed or stacked lag screw fixation, single lag or positional screw fixation with locking or nonlocking plate fixation, staples, and external fixation. **Fig. 8** displays a postoperative radiograph of the first MTP joint arthrodesis and hardware combined with metatarsal head resections. Pan-MTP joint arthrodesis has recently been described as an option for treating a painful severe rheumatoid forefoot deformity, and is performed through 5 dorsal incisions and is fixated with Steinmann pins.[4]

MTP Joint-Sparing Procedures

The modified Hibbs procedure functions as a joint-sparing procedure via release of the MTP joint contractures by tenotomy and transfer of the proximal aspects of the

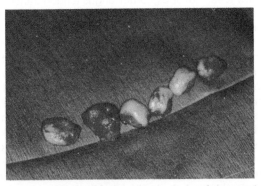

Fig. 7. Five resected metatarsal heads along with the base of the proximal phalanx of the hallux.

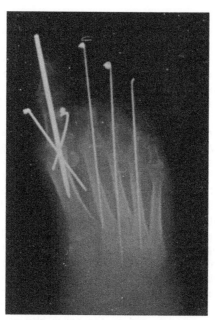

Fig. 8. Postoperative radiograph of first MTP joint arthrodesis and hardware combined with metatarsal head resections.

second, third, and fourth extensor digitorum longus tendons to the dorsolateral midfoot. This is accompanied by the tenotomy and transfer of the proximal aspects of the second, third and fourth extensor digitorum brevis tendons to the remaining distal portion of the extensor digitorum longus tendons of the second, third, and fourth digits, combined with a Z-plasty lengthening of the fifth extensor digitorum longus tendon or anastomosis of the fifth and fourth extensor digitorum longus tendons. **Fig. 9** displays the intraoperative Hibbs incision and the related exposed extensor tendons. Additional joint-sparing procedures that are used to rebalance soft tissues include percutaneous tendon lengthening of the extensor hallucis longus tendon,

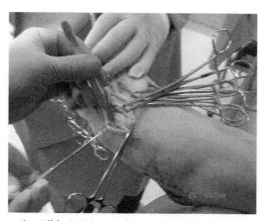

Fig. 9. The intraoperative Hibbs incision and the related exposed extensor tendons.

MTP joint release, extensor hood release, extensor tenotomy or Z-plasty tendon lengthening, capsulotomy, transection of the medial and lateral collateral ligaments, and plantar metatarsal head soft-tissue release via a McGlamry elevator followed by Kirschner wire fixation.[36] The soft-tissue joint-sparing MTP release procedures may be combined with hammertoe or claw toe correction via open, percutaneous, or closed reduction of the digital deformities, followed by Kirschner wire fixation spanning the distal interphalangeal joint, proximal interphalangeal joint and MTP joints. Metatarsal shortening osteotomies provide a joint-sparing bony reconstructive surgical option for the rheumatoid foot. The Weil metatarsal osteotomies with single dorsal to planter screw fixation have been presented as joint-sparing alternatives to the metatarsal head resections, arthroplasties, and first MTP joint arthrodesis procedures.[42] Shortening of the lesser metatarsals may also be combined with fusion or implant arthroplasty of the first MTP joint as well as with open, percutaneous, or closed reduction of digital contractures. Care should be taken to preserve the metatarsal parabola so that the length of the metatarsals reflects a 2, 1, 3, 4, 5 length pattern, with the second metatarsal extending most distally followed by the first and then descending medial to lateral approximately 2 mm from the proceeding metatarsal.[36] The metatarsal shortening point as described by Barouk and Barouk[42] may also be used as a template method for planning and providing the location of the metatarsal shorting osteotomies. Additional first metatarsal osteotomies, such as the Reverdin-Todd, Distal L, and Youngswick osteotomies, should be considered as they may be selectively used to reduce the hallux abducto valgus deformity by reducing the proximal articular set angle, reduce the hallux abductus angle, and reduce the first intermetatarsal angle as well as decompress the joint by shortening the first metatarsal. In the presence of the first intermetatarsal angle being greater than 14°, a proximal first ray procedure such as the Lapidus bunionectomy may be considered, in combination with first metatarsal cuneiform hypermobility and divergence of the dorsal cortex of the first and second metatarsals, to correct the sagittal and transverse plane deformities; or the scarf bunionectomy may be considered in the absence of hypermobility. **Fig. 10** displays a Lapidus procedure with plate and screw fixation as well as an oval to round lucency in the calcaneus depicting the site of a percutaneous calcaneal graft harvest.

Combination of Joint-Destructive and Joint-Sparing Procedures

Historical literature yields to joint-destructive procedures with the Hoffman procedure being favored over the Clayton procedure, probably because of the destabilization of

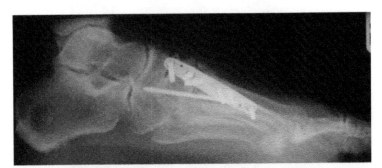

Fig. 10. Lapidus procedure involving plate and screw fixation as well as an oval to round lucency in the calcaneus along with the site of a percutaneous calcaneal graft harvest.

the MTP joint after resection of the base of the proximal phalanxes. Conventional thinking yields to the combination of a first MTP joint arthrodesis with resections of metatarsal heads 2, 3, 4, and 5. The first MTP joint arthrodesis is a viable option when presented with severe hallux abducto valgus, and it is preferred by the surgical authors over resection arthroplasty if the bone stock is adequate for fixation. However, recently the practice of using joint-sparing procedures for rheumatoid forefoot reconstruction is being recognized as a reliable option.[42] The modified Hoffman procedure may also be combined with joint-sparing first MTP joint procedures, such as the first metatarsal osteotomies aimed at correction of hallux abducto valgus and first metatarsal shortening osteotomies. When the emphasis is on surgical reconstruction there is a shift from forefoot joint-destructive procedures to the incorporation of joint-sparing procedures, and therefore a migration to combined procedures that provide the desired benefits of specific joint-destructive and joint-sparing procedures. The inclusion of forefoot joint preservation procedures yields options for combinations of MTP joint-sparing techniques, such as the pan-metatarsal shortening osteotomies, first metatarsal osteotomies, and the Lapidus procedure, with joint-sparing digital MTP joint contracture reduction via soft-tissue releases and tendon balancing procedures such as the modified Hibbs with or without open flexor digitorum longus tendon transfers, percutaneous flexor digital tendonotomies and capsulotomies, or closed digital reduction and Kirschner wire fixation of the distal interphalangeal joint, proximal interphalangeal joint, and MTP joints. **Fig. 11** displays an anteroposterior view of the modified Lapidus and modified Hibbs procedure with intact hardware. The forefoot joint-sparing surgical combination of the modified Lapidus with 3 point 4.0 fully threaded cortical screw fixation, modified Hibbs and digital joint-sparing percutaneous flexor digitorum longus tenotomies, and plantar digital capsulotomies with Kirschner wire fixation address the first ray pathology of hypermobility and hallux

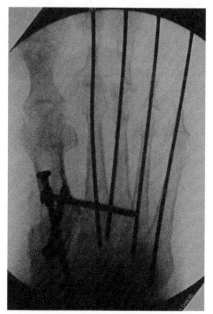

Fig. 11. Anteroposterior view of the modified Lapidus and modified Hibbs procedure with intact hardware.

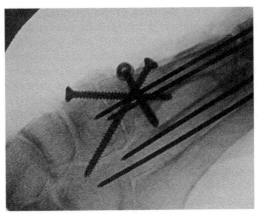

Fig. 12. Lateral view of a modifed Lapidus procedure and modified Hibbs procedure with intact fixation and the resulting sagittal plane correction of the first metatarsal.

abducto valgus while also addressing the lesser digital and MTP joint contracture pathologies. A percutaneous calcaneal bone graft harvest is often performed and used as a sheer-strain relief graft at the first metatarsalcuneiform arthrodesis site.[43] **Fig. 12** displays a lateral view of a modified Lapidus procedure and modified Hibbs procedure with intact fixation, and the resulting sagittal plane correction of the first metatarsal. Open flexor digitorum longus tendon transfers provide a joint-sparing option for reduction of severe hammertoes and aid in the reduction of plantar forefoot pressure and calluses by reducing the retrograde force placed on the metatarsal heads by contracted digits. A percutaneous tendo Achilles lengthening or gastrocnemius recession may also be required in cases where gastrocsoleus equinus or gastrocnemius equinus is present and noted to contribute to excessive plantar forefoot pressure, calluses, or ulceration.[44,45] The surgical authors' reasoning behind choosing a particular approach to reconstructive forefoot surgery in the rheumatoid patient includes avoiding forefoot joint-destructive procedures; stabilizing the first ray without sacrificing first metatarsal joint mobility; releasing joint contractures and providing soft tissue and tendon rebalancing; alleviating the need to entirely reproduce a near anatomic metatarsal parabola as required with resection of the metatarsal heads or shorting osteotomies of the metatarsals; avoiding the risk of delayed union, malunion, and nonunion of the metatarsal osteotomies and MTP arthrodesis procedures; avoiding the potential for development of synovitis associated with failed silicone implants as well as revision of failed implant arthroplasties; nullifiying the potential for distal heterotrophic bone growth post MTP head resection arthroplasties; reducing the expense associated with pan-metatarsal osteotomies and multiple screw fixation while reducing the number of potential screw fixation complications associated with osteoporotic bone; allowing for intramedullary Kirschner wire fixation and temporary stabilization post reduction of the digital and lesser MTP joint contractures without the potential interference of proximal screw fixation associated with lesser metatarsal shortening osteotomies, and because Kirschner wire fixation is less costly than digital screw and digital intramedullary locking fixation.

SUMMARY

Although no one specific test or finding provides a definitive diagnosis of RA, correlation of the clinical, laboratory, radiographic, and MRI findings if available assist in making the diagnosis. Care must be taken to adequately work up a patient with RA before executing elective surgical intervention, and a multidisciplinary team approach including the patient's rheumatologist is recommended during the perioperative phase. Multiple surgical options exist to address the rheumatoid forefoot, such as joint-destructive resection arthroplasties, implant arthroplasties, and arthrodesis procedures; joint-sparing osteotomies, tenotomies, capsulotomies, and tendon transfers; as well as the combination of such joint-sparing and joint-destructive procedures. First metatarsal and lesser metatarsal joint-destructive and joint-sparing procedures with digital joint-destructive and joint-sparing procedures have been presented and opinions have been published regarding the level of evidence and grades of recommendations for several of the procedures.[18] It is the surgical authors' position that most joint-sparing and joint-destructive procedures presented are useful given the appropriate patient and pathology. However, in reviewing the different procedures the authors would highlight the reconstructive forefoot procedures that are joint-sparing and their combination with joint-destructive procedures that stabilize the first ray, as this has been reported to be the key to reconstruction of the rheumatoid forefoot.[8,17] The surgical authors have found the combination of a modified Lapidus bunionectomy with a modified Hibbs procedure and a percutaneous release of digital contractures or an open flexor digitorum longus tendon transfer to provide an effective means for reconstruction of the forefoot in the patient with RA that is both forefoot joint-sparing and first ray stabilizing. At present the surgical authors are not aware of prior publication combining the forefoot joint-sparing and midfoot joint-destructive Lapidus procedure with the forefoot joint-sparing modified Hibbs procedure with the additional digital joint-sparing percutaneous flexor digitorum longus tenotomies, proximal interphalangeal joint capsulotomies and, if needed, distal interphalangeal joint capsulotomies for the reconstruction of the rheumatoid foot, and hence present this combination procedure as another option for the foot and ankle surgeon to consider when surgically reconstructing the foot in the rheumatoid patient.

REFERENCES

1. Pincus T. Rheumatoid arthritis. Common rheumatic diseases. In: Wegener ST, Belza BL, Gall EP, editors. Clinical care in the rheumatic diseases. Georgia (GA): American College of Rheumatology; 1996. p. 147–55.
2. Pincus T, Wolfe F, Callahan LF. Updating a reassessment of traditional paradigms concerning rheumatoid arthritis. In: Wolf F, Pincus T, editors. Rheumatoid arthritis: pathogenesis, assessment, outcome, and treatment. New York: Marcel Dekker Inc; 1994. p. 1–74.
3. Harris ED Jr. Rheumatoid arthritis: pathophysiology and implications for therapy. N Engl J Med 1990;322:1277–89.
4. Jeffries LC, Rodriguez RH, Stapleton JJ, et al. Pan-metatarsophalangeal joint arthrodesis for the severe rheumatoid forefoot deformity. Clin Podiatr Med Surg 2009;26:149–57.
5. Silman AJ, Pearson JE. Epidemiology and genetics of rheumatoid arthritis. Arthritis Res 2002;4(Suppl 3):S265–72.
6. Kadenbande S, Debnath U, Kharana A, et al. Rheumatoid forefoot reconstruction: first metatarsophalangeal fusion and excision arthroplasty of lesser metatarsal heads. Acta Orthop Belg 2007;73(1):88–95.
7. Jen CL. Rheumatoid arthritis in foot and ankle surgery. Foot Ankle Clin 2007;12: xii–v.

8. Stevens BW, Anderson JG, Bohay DR. Hallux metatarsophalangeal fusion for the rheumatoid forefoot by Stevens, in rheumatoid arthritis in foot ankle surgery. Foot Ankle Clin 2007;12(3):395–404.

9. Weinfeld S, Schon L. Hallux metatarsophalangeal arthritis. Clin Orthop Relat Res 1998;349:9–19.

10. Jaakkola JI, Mann RA. A review of rheumatoid arthritis affecting the foot and ankle. Foot Ankle Int 2004;25(12):866–74.

11. Wilder RL. Rheumatoid arthritis. Epidemiology, pathology and pathogenesis. In: Schumacher H, Klippel J, Koopman W, editors. Primer on the rheumatic diseases. 11th edition. Georgia: The Arthritis Foundation; 1997. p. 155–60.

12. Firestein GS, Paine MM, Littman BH. Gene expression (collagenase, tissue inhibition of metalloproteinases, complement, and HLA-DR) in a rheumatoid arthritis and osteopathrosis synovium. Quantitative analysis and effect of intraarticular corticosteroids. Arthritis Rheum 1991;34(9):1094–105.

13. Lawrence RC, Hochberg MC, Kelsy JL. Estimates of the prevalence of selected arthritic and musculoskeletal diseases in the United States. J Rheumatol 1989; 16(4):427–41.

14. Reize P, Leichtle CI, Leichtle UG, et al. Long-term results after metatarsal head resection in the treatment of rheumatoid arthritis. Foot Ankle Int 2006;27(8): 586–90.

15. Fuhrmann R, Abramowski I, Venbrocks R. Spatergenbnisse nach Operationen am rheumatischen Vorfuss und Analyse der Fehlschlage [Late results after surgery on the rheumatoid forefoot and analysis of the failure]. Akt Rheumatol 1995;20:227–33 [in German].

16. Coughlin MJ. Rheumatoid forefoot reconstruction. A long-term follow-up study. J Bone Joint Surg Am 2000;82(3):322–41.

17. Vainio K. Rheumatoid foot. Clinical study with pathological and roentgenological comments. Ann Chir Gynaecol Fenn Suppl 1956;45(1):1–107.

18. Jeng C, Campbell J. Current concepts review. The rheumatoid forefoot. Foot Ankle Int 2008;29(9):959–68.

19. Arnett FC, Edworthy SM, Bloch DA, et al. The American Rheumatism Association 1987 revised criteria for the classification of rheumatoid arthritis. Arthritis Rheum 1988;31:315–24.

20. Molloy AP, Myerson MS. Surgery of the lesser toes in rheumatoid arthritis: metatarsal head resection. Foot Ankle Clin 2007;12:417–33.

21. Brower AC. Arthritis in black and white. Philadelphia: WB Saunders; 1988.

22. Mitchell DM, Spitz PW. Survival prognosis and causes of death in rheumatoid arthritis. Arthritis Rheum 1986;27(2):706–14.

23. Nassar J. Complications of surgery of the foot and ankle in patients with rheumatoid arthritis. Clin Orthop 2001;391:140–52.

24. Mann RA. Management of foot and ankle in rheumatoid arthritis. Rheum Dis Clin North Am 1996;22:457–76.

25. Glynn MK. The significance of asymptomatic bacteruria in patients undergoing hip, knee arthroplasty. Clin Orthop 1984;185:151–4.

26. Clark CR. Rheumatoid involvement of cervical spine an overview. Spine 1994;19: 2257–8.

27. Skues MA, Welchew EA. Anesthesia and rheumatoid arthritis. Anesthesia 1993; 48:989–97.

28. Frank ST, Weg JG. Pulmonary dysfunction in rheumatoid disease. Chest 1973;63: 27–34.

29. Sany J, Anaya JM. Influence of MTX on frequency of postop infectious complications in patients with rheumatoid arthritis. J Rheumatol 1993;20:1129.
30. Perhala RS, Wilke WS. Local infectious complications following large joint replacement in rheumatoid arthritis treated with MTX versus those not treated with MTX. Arthritis Rheum 1991;34:146.
31. Kelley JT, Conn DL. Perioperative management of the rheumatic disease patient. Bull Rheum Dis 2002;51(6):1–7.
32. Lipsky P. Rheumatoid arthritis. In: Kasper D, editor. Harrison's principles of internal medicine. New York: McGraw-Hill; 2005. p. 1968.
33. Bibbo C, Anderson RB, Davis WH, et al. Rheumatoid nodules and postoperative complications. Foot Ankle Int 2003;24(1):40–4.
34. Soter NA, Franks AG. Cutaneous manifestations of rheumatic diseases. In: Kelly WN, Harris ED, Ruddy S, et al, editors. Textbook of rheumatology. 5th edition. Philadelphia: WB Saunders, Premarin, Provera; 1997. p. 497–510.
35. Klippel JH, editor. Appendix I. Primer on the rheumatic diseases. 11th edition. Atlanta (GA): Arthritis Foundation; 1997. p. 454.
36. McGlamry ED, Banks AS, Downey MS. Principles of muscle-tendon surgery and tendon transfers. In: McGlamry ED, Banks AS, Downey MS, editors, Comprehensive textbook of foot surgery, vol. 2. 2nd edition. Baltimore (MD): Willims & Wilkins; 1992. p. 1319–20.
37. Hibbs RA. An operation for "clawfoot. JAMA 1919;73:1583.
38. Clayton ML. Surgery of the forefoot in rheumatoid arthritis. Clin Orthop 1960;16: 136–40.
39. Clayton ML, Leidhold JD, Clark W. Arthroplasty of rheumatoid metatarsophalangeal joints an outcome study. Clin Orthop 1997;340:48–57.
40. Hoffman P. An operation for severe grades of contracted or clawed toes. Am J Orthop Surg 1912;9:441–9.
41. Thomas S, Kinninmonth AWG, Kumar CS. Long-term results of the modified Hoffman procedure with K-wire fixation Procedure in the rheumatoid forefoot. J Bone Joint Surg Am 2006;88:149–57.
42. Barouk LS, Barouk P. Joint-preserving surgery in rheumatoid forefoot: preliminary study with more-than-two-year follow-up. Foot Ankle Clin 2007;12:435–54.
43. DiDomenico LA, Haro AA. Percutaneous harvest of calcaneal graft. J Foot Ankle Surg 2006;45:131–3.
44. Haro AA, DiDomenico LA. Frontal plane-guided percutaneous tendo Achilles' lengthening. J Foot Ankle Surg 2007;46:55–61.
45. DiDomenico LA, Adams HB, Garchar D. Endoscopic gastrocnemius recession for treatment of gastrocnemius equinus. J Am Podiatr Med Assoc 2005;95(4): 410–3.

The Surgical Reconstruction of Rheumatoid Midfoot and Hindfoot Deformities

Jason D. Neufeld, DPM[a,b], Glen M. Weinraub, DPM, FACFAS[c,d,e,*],
Ernesto S. Hernandez, DPM[a,c], Marc S. Co, DPM[a,b]

KEYWORDS

• Rheumatoid arthritis • Midfoot • Hindfoot • Arthrodesis

Rheumatoid arthritis (RA) is a systemic inflammatory disease that predominantly manifests in the synovial membrane of diarthrodial joints.[1] This affliction affects all ethnicities worldwide, particularly those between their fourth and sixth decades.[1] RA can present in either gender, but more commonly affects women than men, at a ratio of 3:1.[2] The criteria for classification of RA are based on clinical evaluation, radiographic examination, and laboratory testing. Depending on the precision of these criteria, it has been estimated that between 0.3% and 1.5% of the North American population is afflicted with this disease.[1]

PATHOPHYSIOLOGY

RA is a chronic and progressive inflammatory disease with unknown cause. Systemic features are associated with RA in most patients, but it is primarily characterized by synovitis and severe joint destruction. Because it destroys the joint synovium, the disease has been termed cancer of the synovial tissues in some modern literature.[2]

---

[a] Kaiser Hayward PMS-36 Residency Program, Hayward, CA, USA
[b] Department of Orthopaedic Surgery, Kaiser Permanente Medical Group, Hayward/Fremont California, 3555 Whipple Road, Building A, Union City, CA 94587, USA
[c] Department of Orthopaedic Surgery, Kaiser Permanente Medical Group, Hayward/Fremont California, 39400 Paseo Padre Parkway, Fremont, CA 94538, USA
[d] Midwestern University School of Podiatric Medicine, Phoenix, AZ, USA
[e] GME Kaiser Permanente GSAA, CA, USA
* Corresponding author. Department of Orthopaedic Surgery, Kaiser Permanente Medical Group, Hayward/Fremont California, 39400 Paseo Padre Parkway, Fremont, CA 94538.
E-mail address: gweinraub@aol.com

Clin Podiatr Med Surg 27 (2010) 261–273
doi:10.1016/j.cpm.2009.12.001
0891-8422/10/$ – see front matter © 2010 Elsevier Inc. All rights reserved.

The synovium is an important source of nutrients for cartilage because cartilage itself is avascular. Typically, a healthy synovium is 1 to 3 cells thick.[2] RA has a complex pathogenesis involving synovial cell proliferation and pannus formation, ending in cartilage and bone destruction. There are theories that the proliferation of RA is initiated by interactions between helper T cells and an unidentified antigen.[2] Once the T cells or CD4+ cells are activated within the joint, there is in turn an activation of macrophages and fibroblasts that is mediated by an interdependent network of cytokines and proteolytic enzymes. The major proinflammatory macrophage-derived cytokines that are expressed in RA synovium and synovial fluid are interleukin 1 (IL-1) and tumor necrosis factor α.[2] IL-1 has a broad range of activities within the RA joint. IL-1 is believed to be the major contributor to the painful inflammatory nature of RA. IL-1 stimulates synoviocytes, chondrocytes, and osteoblasts, with each cell type exhibiting a destructive effect within the RA joint.[2]

Initially, IL-1 mediates inflammation by recruitment of neutrophils into the joint, and activation of macrophages, and further stimulation of T and B cells. IL-1 affects the synovium with proliferation of fibroblasts, which in turn leads to pannus formation. IL-1 also activates chondrocytes to secrete proteolytic enzymes that contribute to the destruction of the joint's own cartilage matrix.[2] This leads to the progressive narrowing of the joint. Osteoblasts are stimulated to differentiate into osteoclasts by IL-1, which in turn leads to increased bone resorption activity and further joint destruction. The tissue repair process is also impaired by prevention of cartilage matrix formation.[2] A complex network of many proinflammatory entities mediates the inflammatory process, but IL-1 is one of the most recognized.

The radiographic features of this disease correlate well with the histopathologic changes. Normal synovium is anchored to both sides of the joint. The hypertrophied rheumatoid synovium begins its invasion of bone at these sites of attachment, which is seen radiographically as erosions on either side of the joint.[3] In addition to bone erosion, the height of cartilage is progressively and symmetrically reduced, consistent with the destructive process of the disease.

CLINICAL PRESENTATION

RA initially presents as foot and ankle symptoms in 20% of cases. Eventually, 50% to 90% of patients develop foot and ankle alterations.[4] Vainio[5] reported a 91% prevalence of foot and ankle symptoms in female rheumatoid patients and 85% in male patients in an inpatient setting, whereas Michelson and colleagues[6] noted a 94% prevalence of foot and ankle symptoms in an outpatient setting.

RA can affect any joint in the foot or ankle without any predictable disease progression. Jaakkola and Mann[7] note that early in the course of RA the forefoot is the most common site of involvement in the lower extremity. Fleming and colleagues[8] reported that the site of onset of RA was the foot in 13% of patients and the ankle in 6% of patients who had had RA for less than a year. Michelson and colleagues[6] reported that ankle and hindfoot symptoms (42%) were more prevalent than forefoot symptoms (28%) in a series of 99 patients followed in an outpatient setting. Other studies[6,9,10] have shown the prevalence of midfoot and hindfoot symptoms is about half that of forefoot and ankle symptoms.

Michelson and colleagues[6] identified the most common features of RA presentation in the foot and ankle. Bilaterality of symptoms predominated in the joints that were studied. Typical deformities of the forefoot include hallux valgus (91%) and hammer toes (94%). Dorsolateral dislocation of the lesser metatarsophalangeal joints results in the hallmark fibular deviation of the digits. Distal migration of the forefoot plantar fat pad secondary to severe hammer toes may result in plantar prominence of the metatarsal heads. Flattening of the medial longitudinal arch, marked abduction of the forefoot on the rearfoot, and heel eversion contribute to increased loading of the medial ligaments and tendons. RA involvement of the hindfoot frequently leads to planovalgus deformity. Michelson and colleagues[6] identified pes planus in 64% of patients with RA. In addition, 34% of the 196 ankles tested exhibited limited range of motion (ROM), which contributed to pain in 23% of ankles.

Soft-tissue manifestations include synovitis, bursitis, tendinitis, fasciitis, neuritis, and vasculitis.[11] Although any tendon can be symptomatic, the posterior tibial tendon (PTT) has received the most attention. Hindfoot valgus and pes planus are common findings in patients with RA, but controversy exists whether the deformity is caused by PTT dysfunction (PTTD) or ligamentous laxity secondary to RA.[6,10,12,13] Of the 64% occurrence of pes planus, Michelson and colleagues[6] determined that 11% had PTTD based on physical examination. However, others have stated that the valgus deformity of the hindfoot is caused by tarsal joint arthritis or subtalar joint (STJ) inflammation, which leads to ligamentous laxity and PTT weakness.[14] Whether ligamentous or tendinous structures are primarily involved, loading of these static and dynamic soft-tissue structures contributes to the rheumatoid flatfoot.

Another common soft-tissue lesion found in patients with RA is the rheumatoid nodule. These nodules typically are firm, nontender, and movable masses measuring up to 5 cm. They often occur on extensor surfaces and in areas of increased pressure, such as the medial and lateral malleoli and the medial and lateral eminences of the forefoot.[7] Neurologic involvement can be a generalized neuropathy, but tarsal tunnel syndrome or an interdigital neuroma may occur. Proposed causes include compression from rheumatoid nodules, synovitic tissue, tenosynovitis, vascular lesions, and valgus deformity.[5,11,15]

IMAGING

Because the early pathologic changes of RA are nonosseous in nature, magnetic resonance imaging (MRI) has been shown to be superior to conventional radiography and computed tomography (CT) as a diagnostic tool. Inflammatory changes such as hyperemia, synovitis, and joint effusion are first detected on MRI before radiographic evidence.[16] Hetland and colleagues[17,18] found that MRI was the strongest predictor of subsequent radiographic progression in early RA. There is no general consensus on which joints to image. Joints typically involved in RA, such as wrist and hand joints, are usually imaged. Michelson and colleagues[6] report that lower extremity joints are affected earlier in the disease process than upper extremity joints. When the foot and ankle are the initial complaint, MRI imaging of symptomatic joints may also be used in the early detection of RA. MRI has become the standard for visualization of nonosseous pathologic processes early in the disease course. Medical management of the autoimmune and inflammatory pathways can then be initiated after MRI aids diagnosis.

Osseous changes, which may be sequelae of the chronic inflammatory process, are typically evaluated with conventional radiography and CT. Radiographic examination routinely includes weight-bearing anteroposterior, lateral, and medial oblique views of the foot and anteroposterior, lateral, and anterior mortise views of the ankle. Systematically, the ankle and foot joints should be evaluated for periarticular soft-tissue swelling, symmetric narrowing of the joint space, marginal cortical erosions, osteoporosis, and subchondral cysts. Localized involvement of the metatarsophalangeal, talonavicular (TN), naviculocuneiform, calcaneocuboid (CC), or ankle joint may be present, although any joint may exhibit osseous changes associated with RA pathology.

When evaluating a patient with rheumatoid pes planus deformity that is being considered for surgical intervention, it is imperative to determine the origin of the deformity. A lateral radiograph helps to determine the level of the deformity. Subluxation of the TN joint is often seen in the rheumatoid flatfoot. Collapse of this joint causes a rearfoot valgus deformity. An anteroposterior ankle radiograph must be viewed to make sure that the valgus deformity of the rearfoot is not secondary to an ankle valgus deformity.

MIDFOOT ARTHRITIS

In combination with hindfoot symptoms, midfoot symptoms represent around half of all forefoot and ankle symptoms.[6,10] A high rate of midfoot involvement has been shown radiographically. Vidigal and colleagues[10] described radiographic evidence of RA in the tarsometatarsal (TMT) joints of 62% of 204 feet. Of this 62%, only 27% of patients were symptomatic in the TMT joint. However, often it is not the rheumatoid synovitis that leads to symptoms in these areas but hindfoot valgus and hallux valgus deformities that increase weight-bearing stresses across the midfoot joints.[7]

Spiegel and Spiegel[13] found that flattening of the longitudinal arch occurred in approximately 50% of patients with chronic RA. On lateral weight-bearing radiographs, sagging at either the metatarsocuneiform or the naviculocuneiform articulation demonstrates this loss of the longitudinal arch and resultant rocker bottom deformity. Concomitantly, first TMT dorsiflexion and lesser toe TMT abduction and dorsiflexion are further resulting deformities with disease progression.[7] Eventually, in the chronic disease state, chronic synovitis and resultant chrondrolysis occur at the TMT joints. A fibrous or bony ankylosis ensues on further progression of the disease because of the limitation of motion at the midfoot joints.[19]

HINDFOOT ARTHRITIS

Hindfoot (STJ, TN, and CC joints) involvement in patients with RA increases with a longer duration of disease.[7,20] The pathophysiology behind hindfoot involvement involves a progressive destruction of the capsular and ligamentous structures that encompass the STJ.[19] Because of the intimate relationship between the STJ and the metatarsal joint, instability at 1 of these joints leads to altered function and gait and increases the likelihood of progression to a pes planovalgus deformity of the hindfoot. Cracchiolo[20] reinforced this idea by stating that "synovitis of the hindfoot joints, subsequent loss of articular cartilage, erosion of the subtalar joints and possible posterior tendon dysfunction can lead to a persistent valgus deformity of the hindfoot that is seen in approximately 80% patients with hindfoot involvement." In addition, Downey and colleagues[21] looked at the relationship between PTTD in RA and the unilateral progressive flatfoot deformities seen in these patients and found them to be intimately related. Spiegel and Spiegel[13] reported that only 8% patients who had had disease for less than 5 years had moderate to severe hindfoot deformities, whereas of those patients who had had RA for more than 5 years, 25% had abnormal hindfoot valgus on weight bearing.

CONSERVATIVE TREATMENT

In the conservative management of midfoot and hindfoot RA there are various treatment modalities, all limited in effectiveness by the severity of the disease process.

Options include rest to relieve edematous and inflamed joints and limiting weight bearing during acute flares of the disease. In addition, padding, casting, roomy shoes, soft orthosis, University of California Biomechanics Laboratory insert, and custom foot orthoses can all help alleviate symptoms and disease progression.[7] When there is a significant amount of instability, ankle-foot orthosis can provide some additional benefit. Symptomatic relief can also be obtained by judicious use of corticosteroid injections and nonsteroidal antiinflammatory drugs.[19,22]

PREOPERATIVE ASSESSMENT

The preoperative examination for rheumatoid patients must include timing of the procedure and medication management with appropriate consultation to ensure a desirable operative and postoperative course. The precise timing for surgical intervention in the rheumatoid foot must be individualized for each patient, as the disease process varies from patient to patient. In this regard, it is best to consult the patient's rheumatologist to review the treatment plan to minimize postoperative morbidity.

When evaluating the rheumatoid patient's medication list, special attention needs to be paid to the rheumatologic agents, as improper perioperative management of these medications can lead to various complications. Disease-modifying antirheumatic agents have been shown to cause delays in wound healing, infection, and bone marrow suppression. It has been recommended that methotrexate be withheld for 1 to 2 weeks before surgery in patients with renal disease. However, in patients with normal renal function there is no reason to stop perioperative methotrexate.[23] Prednisone has been associated with postoperative complications like nonunions and delays in wound healing, in patients taking more than 7.5 mg/d.[24] Nonsteroidal antiinflammatory agents can increase intraoperative and postoperative bleeding. Consultation with the patient's rheumatologist is prudent before prescribing a perioperative medication plan.

In addition, a clinical and radiographic assessment of the cervical spine should be performed in those patients who are about to undergo an operation under general or spinal anesthesia. To assess the stability of the neck, lateral views with the cervical spine in neutral, flexion, and extension are beneficial.[20]

SURGICAL INTERVENTION

When conservative care no longer tempers the patient's symptoms, surgical intervention should be the next step. The indications for arthrodesis of the involved joints include pain, instability, deformity that does not allow normal joint function, and failure of joint-sparing or replacement surgeries.

TMT ARTHRODESIS

The TMT joint has classically been divided into 3 compartments. Making up the medial column is the first metatarsal and medial cuneiform. The second and third metatarsals with the middle and lateral cuneiforms make up the middle column, and the lateral column is composed of the fourth and fifth metatarsals and the cuboid. The medial column is the most mobile, followed by the lateral column. Because of the keystone effect of the second metatarsal as it extends further proximal than any of the other metatarsals, the middle column is left with little motion.[25–27]

If the TN joint is categorized as a hindfoot joint, then the first metatarsocuneiform joint is the most commonly affected joint of the midfoot in RA. Involvement of this medial column joint can lead to collapse of the medial longitudinal arch. According to Jaakkola and Mann,[7] symptoms in the first TMT joint are often not caused by rheumatoid synovitis, but by valgus deformities of the hindfoot and hallux that increase stress across this area. With the exception of the medial column, the middle and lateral columns of the TMT joint are rarely involved. When there is degenerative joint disease at these levels, it is usually asymptomatic because of the lack of motion in the central and lateral columns. As mentioned earlier, it is usually degeneration secondary to breakdown and collapse of other joints, instead of rheumatoid synovitis, that leads to arthritic changes in these areas.

Arthrodesis of the first metatarsocuneiform joint has been used successfully in stabilizing the medial arch. However, more commonly, it has been used to fuse the first metatarsocuneiform joint in RA patients with severe hallux valgus deformities. Lapidus[28,29] first mainstreamed this procedure for its use with primary metatarsal primus adductus with hallux valgus. Recent studies have shown that the modified Lapidus arthrodesis not only corrects hallux valgus deformities and stabilizes the medial arch but also helps improve the medial longitudinal arch height. Avino and colleagues[30] found that Meary angle and medial cuneiform height improved significantly, on average 2.97° and 3.44 mm, respectively, following modified Lapidus arthrodesis.

Operative management largely involves arthrodesis of the involved TMT joints. It can be difficult to determine which joints to arthrodese. The increased overlap of the TMT joints on radiographs, difficulty in isolating ROM in this joint complex, and the patient's inability to locate areas of pain or discomfort precisely all lead to complicated determinations of the level of disease. Diagnostic imaging besides radiographs, such as bone scans and CT, can aid the foot and ankle surgeon's accurate diagnosis of the extent of TMT involvement. The cuboid should not be fused to the lateral column, even if the fourth and fifth TMT joints are affected, because these joints are often asymptomatic and help maintain flexibility.[27]

Many different fixation techniques have been used successfully for TMT arthrodesis, including Kirschner wire, screw, combination of screws and plates (**Fig. 1**), and staple fixation. It is important for the surgeon to determine whether a realignment arthrodesis is necessary versus an in situ arthrodesis. If deformity at the TMT joint is determined then realignment of the rheumatoid foot is indicated. When only single joint involvement with little deformity is seen, then in situ arthrodesis is appropriate.[7]

CC ARTHRODESIS

Isolated arthritis of the CC joint in a patient with RA is rare and is predominantly the result of medial longitudinal arch collapse and abnormal motion across the STJ and midtarsal joint.[27] An isolated CC joint arthrodesis is atypical outside posttraumatic conditions involving this joint. This procedure is often combined with a TN arthrodesis or part of the triple arthrodesis procedure. Clain and Baxter[31] advocated the use of the double arthrodesis (TN and CC joints) in cases of isolated TN arthritis and peritalar subluxation in RA.

NAVICULOCUNEIFORM ARTHRODESIS

The naviculocuneiform joint along with the CC, intercuneiform, and medial TMT joints have been defined as nonessential joints for normal gait.[32,33] Thus, the naviculocuneiform joint can be sacrificed to allow stability of the medial column in pes planovalgus deformities afflicting RA patients without having a significant effect on gait after fusion. First described by Hoke in 1931, the navicular-cuneiform arthrodesis involved fusion of the navicular to the medial and intermediate cuneiforms along with lengthening of

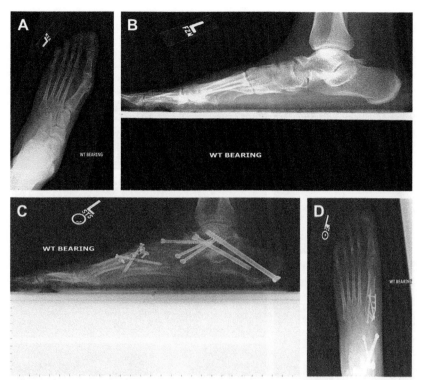

Fig. 1. A 35-year-old man with juvenile RA and middle facet coalition (*A, B*). Compound deformities required Lapidus and medial approach TN joint and STJ arthrodesis (*C, D*). (*Courtesy of* Glen M. Weinraub, DPM.)

the Achilles tendon. To help restore the medial longitudinal arch in a flatfoot deformity, Hoke[34] removed a plantarly based wedge from the joint and then used an onlay bone graft to bridge the arthrodesis site. RA rarely affects the naviculocuneiform joint primarily, and as the duration of the disease increases the entire medial column can soon be affected (**Fig. 2**). However, if it is the only joint affected, a naviculocuneiform arthrodesis can afford a satisfactory result. Chi and colleagues[32] showed an average decrease in Meary angle and TN coverage of 20° and 10°, respectively in 5 feet that underwent arthrodesis of the naviculocuneiform joint and first metatarsocuneiform joint.

Various techniques have been described for naviculocuneiform arthrodesis, including wedge resections, cartilage resection, and bone-block resection with onlay bone grafting. Specifically with fixation, successful arthrodesis can result from using screws, plates, staples, and external fixators when indicated.[27]

TN ARTHRODESIS

Of all the joints in the hindfoot, the TN articulation is often the first joint to undergo degenerative changes associated with RA.[35] Early radiographic changes include increased soft-tissue edema, narrowing of the joint space, subchondral sclerosis, and peritalar subluxation in a medial and plantar direction. In advanced cases there might be ankylosis with complete collapse of the TN joint architecture.[36] In 1967,

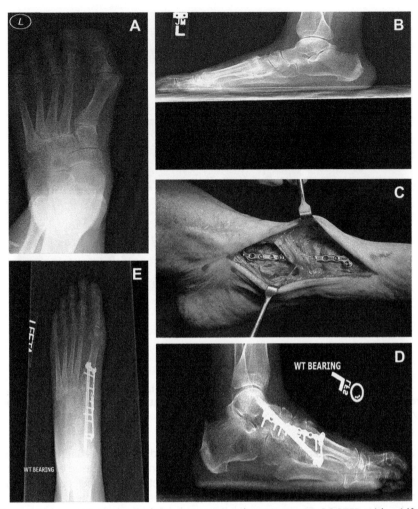

Fig. 2. A 68-year-old woman with long-term RA, subsequent stage 2C PTTD with midfoot changes and hallux abducto valgus (*A, B*). Complete medial column fusion was required. Locking plates are stacked over modified beaming application (*C, D, E*). The patient was doing well at 24-month follow-up. (*Courtesy of* Glen M. Weinraub, DPM.)

Vahvanen[37] found that narrowing of the TN joint space and midfoot collapse consistently occurred within 3 years of the diagnosis of RA.

Indications for isolated arthrodesis of the TN joint in the rheumatoid foot have been discussed in the literature. Elbaor and colleagues[38] believed this isolated fusion was indicated if pain persisted at the TN joint despite an adequate trial of conservative therapy and if a permanent hindfoot valgus deformity had yet to occur. Kindsfater and colleagues[39] supported this concept, stating that for "isolated, painful, talonavicular arthritis with mild deformity, selective arthrodesis of this joint alone seems to be the procedure of choice." Some investigators have deemed this procedure more appropriate for older less active rheumatoid patients and advocated the addition of the CC joint in the arthrodesis in younger more active individuals.[40]

The interrelation of the triple joint complex sets up a natural progression of deformity in RA. Prompt fusion of the TN joint when the indications already mentioned are met can lead to cessation of such pathologic processes. Lapidus[29] highlighted this inter-connectivity in 1955 when he reported that fixing the transverse tarsal joints significantly decreased STJ motion. More recently, Wulker and colleagues[41] found that hindfoot motion was essentially eliminated when the TN joint was fused alone or in combination. Astion and colleagues[42] found that any combination of simulated arthrodesis involving the TN joint limited motion in the CC and STJ to about 2°, respectively. Fusion of the TN joint may obviate fusing the STJ.

Kinsfater and colleagues[39] reported 104 isolated TN fusions from previous studies and found that more than 95% of patients obtained good to excellent pain relief, with a nonunion rate of only 5%. During the mean follow-up period of 52 months no patient required triple arthrodesis for progressive valgus deformity.

STJ ARTHRODESIS

Seltzer and colleagues[43] using CT investigated a series of patients with RA and noted degenerative changes of the STJ in 29%. Other investigators have reported the involvement of the STJ to be between 32% and 42%.[6,10]

Patients with rheumatoid degenerative changes of the STJ commonly present with pain, chronic edema, stiffness, ataxic gait, and difficulty walking on uneven surfaces. A progressive pes planovalgus deformity is often the result of joint collapse from continued weight bearing on this unstable platform.[36]

The decision to perform an isolated arthrodesis of the STJ has elicited controversy. However, if there is only arthritic involvement of the STJ on careful radiographic inspection without concomitant involvement of the midtarsal and ankle joints, and a diagnostic injection into the STJ has provided complete cessation of symptoms, an isolated arthrodesis is warranted. In a retrospective review of isolated subtalar disorders in 11 feet, Mann and Baumgarten[44] found isolated STJ arthrodesis to be a satisfactory method of treatment. Although some patients in their study did develop mild talar beaking and osteophyte formation at the CC joint, these investigators found that the changes were not clinically significant. Functional and pain ratings for the patient population after the isolated STJ arthrodesis were good to excellent.

TRIPLE ARTHRODESIS

Ryerson,[45] in 1923, first coined the term triple arthrodesis when he described an arthrodesis of the subastragaloid (STJ) and mediotarsal (midtarsal) joint. The purpose of this procedure was to correct deformity, relieve pain, stabilize, and achieve a plantigrade foot. This operation is still the preferred method of treatment of complex hindfoot disease, as seen in advanced stages of RA. In the setting of clinical and radiographic evidence of STJ and midtarsal joint arthritis, operative intervention is indicated when there is severe pain that is unresponsive to conservative therapy.

The traditional approach involves using 2 incisions. The medial incision is used to visualize the TN joint and the lateral incision is used to visualize the STJ and CC joint. Recent studies have advocated a single incision medial approach, which has the advantages of reducing operative time, eliminating lateral dissection, and avoiding lateral wound dehiscence in the severe valgus hindfoot.[46,47] This is especially important in rheumatoid patients. To get adequate correction in a long-standing hindfoot valgus deformity, surgeons run the risk of stretching apart the lateral skin incision, making closure and subsequent wound healing difficult in this high-risk patient population when using the traditional 2 incision approach.

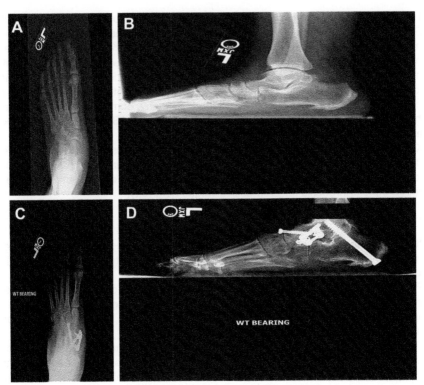

Fig. 3. A 56-year-old woman with RA who developed stage 2C PTTD (*A, B*). She underwent medial approach TN joint and STJ arthrodesis (*C, D*). She was doing well at 18-month follow-up. (*Courtesy of* Glen M. Weinraub, DPM.)

Of all the hindfoot joints, the CC joint has been shown to be the least likely to be involved in the disease process.[43] A double arthrodesis of the TN and STJ can thus spare the uninvolved CC joint while still correcting the pes planovalgus deformity (**Fig. 3**). This in turn avoids potential complications like painful nonunions of the CC joint.[48]

In a recent long-term retrospective review, Knupp and colleagues[49] investigated fusion rates, arthritis of adjacent joints, clinical outcome, and patient satisfaction in 28 patients with RA who had undergone triple arthrodesis. All patients said they would have the same procedure again under similar circumstances. They all went on to radiographic fusion and had an average AOFAS (American Orthopaedic Foot and Ankle Society) score of 70. However, these investigators found a high risk of arthritis in adjacent joints, especially the midfoot joints, after triple arthrodesis.[49] Arthritis of adjacent joints was also more prevalent in a recent cadaver study comparing peak ankle joint pressures after triple arthrodesis and TN arthrodesis, respectively. Suckel and colleagues[50] measured significantly higher peak pressures in the ankle joint after triple arthrodesis than after TN arthrodesis alone.

SUMMARY

RA is a systemic inflammatory disorder that commonly manifests in the joints of the midfoot and hindfoot in the later stages of disease. The varying degrees of joint destruction associated with RA can be severely disabling. Primary arthrodesis, when indicated, of the involved joints has been shown not only to relieve pain but also to allow previously afflicted patients to return to their normal lifestyle.

REFERENCES

1. Goronzy JJ, Weyand CM. Rheumatoid arthritis. In: Klippel JH, editor. Primer on the rheumatic diseases. 12th edition. Atlanta (GA): Arthritis Foundation; 2001. p. 209–32.
2. Koopman W, Moreland L. Arthritis and allied conditions, A textbook of rheumotology. 15th edition. Philadelphia: Lippincott Williams and Wilkins; 2005.
3. Imboden J, Hellmann D, Stone J. Current rheumatology diagnosis and treatments. 2nd edition. New York: McGraw Hill; 2007.
4. Crevoisier X, Assal M. Surgery of the rheumatoid foot and ankle. Rev Med Suisse 2008;4(184):2732–6.
5. Vainio K. Rheumatoid foot. Clinical study with pathological and roentgenological comments. Ann Chir Gynaecol Fenn 1956;45(Suppl):1–107.
6. Michelson J, Easley M, Wigley FM, et al. Foot and ankle problems in rheumatoid arthritis. Foot Ankle 1994;15:608–13.
7. Jaakkola J, Mann R. A review of rheumatoid arthritis affecting the foot and ankle. Foot Ankle Int 2004;25(12):866–74.
8. Fleming A, Crown JM, Corbett M. Early rheumatoid disease. 1. Onset. Ann Rheum Dis 1976;35:357–60.
9. Fuchs HA, Brooks RH, Callahan LF, et al. A simplified twenty-eight-joint quantitative articular index in rheumatoid arthritis. Arthritis Rheum 1989;32:531–7.
10. Vidigal E, Jacoby RK, Dixon AS, et al. The foot in chronic rheumatoid arthritis. Ann Rheum Dis 1975;34:292–7.
11. O'Brien TS, Hart TS, Gould JS. Extraosseous manifestations of rheumatoid arthritis in the foot and ankle. Clin Orthop 1997;340:26–33.
12. Gschwend N, Steiger U. Stable fixation in hindfoot arthrodesis; a valuable procedure in the complex RA foot. In: Schatten-Kirchner M, editor. Rheumatology, vol. 11. Basel, Switzerland: Karger; 1987. p. 114–26.
13. Spiegel TM, Spiegel JS. Rheumatoid arthritis in the foot and ankle – diagnosis, pathology and treatment. Foot Ankle 1982;2:318–24.
14. Keenan MA, Peabody TD, Groley JK, et al. Valgus deformities of the feet and characteristics of gait in patients who have rheumatoid arthritis. J Bone Joint Surg Am 1991;73:237–47.
15. Grabois M, Puentes J, Lidsky M. Tarsal tunnel syndrome in rheumatoid arthritis. Arch Phys Med Rehabil 1981;62:401–3.
16. McQueen F, Benton N, Perry D, et al. Bone edema scored on magnetic resonance imaging scans at presentation of the dominant carpus at presentation predicts radiographic joint damage of the hands and feet six years later in patients with rheumatoid arthritis. Arthritis Rheum 2003;48(7):1814–27.
17. Hetland M, Ejberg B, Horslev-Petersen K, et al. MRI bone edema is the strongest predictor of subsequent radiographic progression in early rheumatoid arthritis. Results from a two year randomized controlled trial (CIMESTRA). Ann Rheum Dis 2009;68:384–90.
18. Haavardsholm E, Boyesen P, Ostergaard M, et al. Magnetic resonance imaging findings in 84 patients with early rheumatoid arthritis: bone marrow edema predicts erosive progression. Ann Rheum Dis 2008;67:794–800.

19. Shurnas PS, Coughlin MJ. Arthritic conditions of the foot. In: Coughlin MJ, Mann RA, Saltzman CL, editors. Surgery of the foot and ankle, 8th edition vol. 1. Philadelphia: Mosby, Inc; 2007. p. 805–921.

20. Cracchiolo A III. Rheumatoid arthritis. Hindfoot disease. Clin Orthop 1997;340: 56–68.

21. Downey DJ, Simkin PA, Mack LA. Tibialis posterior tendon rupture: a cause of rheumatoid flat foot. Arthritis Rheum 1988;31(3):441–6.

22. Smyth CJ, Janson RW. Rheumatologic view of the rheumatoid foot. Clin Orthop Relat Res 1997;340:7–17.

23. Kaczander BI, Cramblett JG, Mann GS. Perioperative management of the podiatric surgical patient. Clin Podiatr Med Surg 2007;24:223–44.

24. Cracchiolo A III, Cimino WR, Lian G. Arthrodesis of the ankle in patients who have rheumatoid arthritis. J Bone Joint Surg Am 1992;74:903–9.

25. Myerson MS. Tarsometatarsal arthrodesis. Foot Ankle 1996;1:73–83.

26. Ouzounian TJ, Shereff MJ. In vitro determination of midfoot motion. Foot Ankle 1989;10:140.

27. Mandracchia VJ, Buddecke DE, Haverstock BD, et al. Evaluation and surgical management of the arthritic midfoot secondary to rheumatic disease. Clin Podiatr Med Surg 1999;16(2):303–26.

28. Lapidus PW. Operative correction of the metatarsus varus primus in hallux valgus. Surg Gynecol Obstet 1934;58:183–91.

29. Lapidus PW. Subtalar joint, its anatomy and mechanics. Bull Hosp Joint Dis 1955; 16:179–95.

30. Avino A, Patel S, Hamilton GA, et al. The effect of the Lapidus arthrodesis on medial longitudinal arch: a radiographic review. J Foot Ankle Surg 2008;47(6): 510–4.

31. Clain MR, Baxter DE. Simultaneous calcaneocuboid and talonavicular fusion: long-term follow-up study. J Bone Joint Surg Br 1994;76:133–6.

32. Chi TD, Toolan BC, Sangeorzan BJ. The lateral column lengthening and medial column stabilization procedures. Clin Orthop 1999;365:81–90.

33. Hansen S. Naviculocuneiform joint arthrodesis. In: Hansen S, editor. Functional reconstruction of the foot and ankle. Philadelphia: Lipincott, Williams & Wilkin; 2007. p. 327–9.

34. Hoke M. An operation for the correction of extremely relaxed flatfeet. J Bone Joint Surg 1931;13:773.

35. Gold RH, Bassett LW. Radiologic evaluation of the arthritic foot. Foot Ankle 1982; 2(6):332–41.

36. Steinberg JS, Hadi SA. Surgical correction of the rearfoot in rheumatoid arthritis. Clin Podiatr Med Surg 1999;16(2):327–36.

37. Vahvanen VA. Rheumatoid arthritis in the pantalar joints: a follow-up study of triple arthrodesis on 292 adult feet. Acta Orthop Scand 1967;107:3.

38. Elbaor MO, Thomas WH, Weinfeld MS, et al. Talonavicular arthrodesis for rheumatoid arthritis of the hindfoot. Orthop Clin North Am 1976;7:821.

39. Kindsfater K, Wilson MG, Thomas WH. Management of the rheumatoid hindfoot with special reference to talonavicular arthrodesis. Clin Orthop Relat Res 1997; 340:69–74.

40. Mann RA, Coughlin MJ. Arthritides. In: Mann RA, Coughlin MJ, editors. Surgery of the foot and ankle. 6th edition. Philadelphia: Mosby; 1993. p. 637.

41. Wulker N, Stukenborg C, Savory KM. Hindfoot motion after isolated and combined arthrodesis: measurements in anatomic specimens. Foot Ankle Int 2000;21(11):921–7.

42. Astion DJ, Deland JT, Otis JC. Motion of the hindfoot after simulated arthrodesis. J Bone Joint Surg Am 1997;79(2):241–6.
43. Seltzer SE, Weissman BN, Braunstein EM, et al. Computed tomography of the hindfoot with rheumatoid arthritis. Arthritis Rheum 1985;28(11):1234–42.
44. Mann RA, Baumgarten M. Subtalar fusion for isolated subtalar disorders. Preliminary report. Clin Orthop Relat Res 1988;226:260–5.
45. Ryerson EW. Arthrodesing operations on the feet. J Bone Joint Surg 1923;5: 453–71.
46. Brilhault J. Single medial approach to modified double arthodesis in rigid flatfoot with lateral deficient skin. Foot Ankle Int 2009;30(1):21–6.
47. Jeng CL, Vora AM, Myerson MS. The medial approach to triple arthrodesis. Indications and technique for management of rigid valgus deformities in high-risk patients. Foot Ankle Clin 2005;10:515–21.
48. Sammarco VJ, Magur EG, Sammarco GJ, et al. Arthrodesis of the subtalar and talonavicular joints for correction of symptomatic hindfoot malalignment. Foot Ankle Int 2006;27:661–6.
49. Knupp M, Skoog A, Tornkvist H, et al. Triple arthrodesis in rheumatoid arthritis. Foot Ankle Int 2008;29(3):293–7.
50. Suckel A, Muller O, Herberts T, et al. Talonavicular arthrodesis or triple arthrodesis: Peak pressure in the adjacent joints measured in 8 cadaver specimens. Acta Orthop 2007;78(5):592–7.

Surgery on the Rheumatoid Ankle Joint: Efficacy Versus Effectiveness

Joseph R. Treadwell, DPM

KEYWORDS

• Rheumatoid arthritis • Synovectomy • Ankle arthrodesis
• Total ankle arthroplasty

Synovectomy, ankle arthrodesis (AA), and total ankle arthroplasty (TAA) are surgical options that address early and late stage diseases in the rheumatoid ankle joint. Synovectomy, for early stage disease, is considered prophylactic at times and is viewed with skepticism because of the chronic inflammatory process within joints that results in progressive tissue degradation and joint destruction. AA and TAA are the 2 most common procedures implemented for symptomatic end-stage joint destruction. The painful ankylosed ankle in patients with rheumatoid arthritis (RA) is one scenario in which the treatment of choice, ankle fusion for end-stage joint destruction, provides an outcome while considered definitive to that specific joint but is not preferred to the maintenance of motion. Total ankle replacement of early generation designs did not provide consistent desired results furthering AA as the treatment of choice. Newer generation ankle implant designs present an opportunity to reassess treatment algorithms for end-stage RA. The progressive disease process associated with RA complicates the long-term outcomes of all treatment options because it has systemic effects on bone, soft tissue, blood vessels, and viscera. The emergence of osteoimmunology provides a greater understanding of the RA disease process. Understanding the pathophysiology of RA gives the surgeon a greater insight as to how this disease can affect procedure outcome. Gait patterns in the patients with RA are significantly altered in end-stage disease as compared with healthy individuals (HI) and should be considered during procedure selection. The effect of RA on bone mineral density (BMD) affects the effectiveness of fixation, and an awareness of the biomechanical differences of various fixation techniques in bones of differing densities is crucial to obtaining stability. This article reviews synovectomy, AA, and associated concepts. A delineation of physiologic interactions associated with RA is provided. TAA is reviewed in the article by DiDomenico and Treadwell elsewhere in this issue.

Foot & Ankle Specialists of Connecticut, PC, 6 Germantown Road, Danbury, CT 06810, USA
E-mail address: jtread6692@aol.com

Clin Podiatr Med Surg 27 (2010) 275–293
doi:10.1016/j.cpm.2009.12.008   **podiatric.theclinics.com**

OSTEOIMMUNOLOGY

An understanding of the physiologic process of RA provides an insight as to how the disease process progresses and affects surgical outcomes. Interactions between the immune system and the skeletal system have led to the development of osteoimmunology. This field of study is particularly relevant to the understanding of RA, as an immune-mediated regulation of bone loss is a well-developed concept that allows for an understanding of the architectural changes in bones that occur within this disease process. Bone remodeling is regulated by molecular and cellular events that coordinate the dynamic balance between osteoblastic and osteoclastic activity.[1] Interference of this balance can result in bone loss as demonstrated in RA.[2] The combination of chronic immune activation and musculoskeletal tissue damage is present in RA.[3] Inflammation is a defining factor in RA especially in the most severe cases. Periarticular bone destruction, a central feature of RA, requires the presence of osteoclasts (OCs) in the joint because this is the only cell type that can remove calcium from bone.[1] OCs are present within the inflamed synovial tissue and the bone-pannus interface in RA.[4] RA is essentially a purely erosive disease with minimal indication of bone repair. The immune and skeletal systems have demonstrated various regulatory molecules in common, such as cytokines.[5] The physiology and pathology of one system affects the other. Because immune cells are formed in the bone marrow by interacting with bone cells, abnormal activation of the immune system can lead to synovial hyperplasia and bone destruction in RA.

The induction of OC precursors near the bone or joint surface to form OCs is mediated by factors in the local environment including within the synovium.[6] When these factors bind to OC precursors multiple genes are expressed that are vital to the function of OCs. As OCs undergo structural changes, they bind to the bone surface, acidify the microenvironment, decalcify the bone, mobilize the mineral content, break down the bone matrix, and then excrete the degradation products into the circulation. These products include solubilized calcium and phosphate, which are intricately involved in maintaining systemic homeostasis.

The expression of receptor activator of nuclear factor-κB ligand (RANKL), also known as osteoclast differentiation factor, osteoprotegerin (OPG) ligand, and tumor necrosis factor-related activation-induced cytokine, has been identified in the synovium of patients with RA, whereas it is not detected in the synovium of patients with other bone diseases.[7] RANKL is an essential stimulating signal for osteoclastogenesis and is involved in the activation of mature OCs.[8] RANKL in connection with macrophage colony-stimulating factor (M-CSF) aids in OC differentiation.

Cytokines are a category of signaling molecules that function extensively in cellular communication. Inflammatory cytokines, such as tumor necrosis factor (TNF)α, interleukin (IL)-1, and IL-6, can act to upregulate or accelerate bone destruction in RA.[9] TNF-α induces RANKL and also stimulates OC precursor cells to synergize with RANKL signaling while inhibiting osteoblasts to affect bone mass locally and systemically.[10] Erosion sites in RA demonstrate pooling of OC precursors in bone marrow cells adjacent to the invading pannus.[7] Synovial tissue in patients with RA is a source of RANKL further implying its involvement in bone erosion.

T-cell infiltration is a hallmark of RA synovium.[11] The bone-lymphocyte relationship has been well appreciated because the early development of lymphocytes occurs in bone. Typically there is no bone loss under normal T-cell response. T cells have an inhibitory effect on osteoclastogenesis via secretion of interferon (IFN)–γ and IL-4 that inhibit RANK and block osteoclastogenesis. However, in vivo studies have demonstrated that T-cell–derived RANKL is responsible for osteoclastogenesis and focal erosion under pathologic conditions, such as RA.[12] Suppression of IFN-γ inhibits its osteoclastic suppression. T-helper (T_H) cells that produce IL-17 (T_H17) have a decisive function in the destruction associated with RA.[13] T_H17 cells have also demonstrated involvement with tissue damage from inflammation and organ-specific autoimmunity. IL-17 has been linked to synovial inflammation and cartilage and bone destruction. IL-17 is spontaneously produced in RA synovium and has a significantly higher concentration in synovial fluid when compared with osteoarthritis (OA) and normal joints.[14]

Whereas T cells express RANKL that influences osteoclastogenesis, B cells have an indirect effect on bone metabolism.[15] Rheumatoid factor (RF) is an autoantibody derived from B cells. RF is an antibody to the Fc portion of the immunoglobulin (Ig)G that is also an antibody. These 2 antibodies form immune complexes that are involved in the pathology associated with RA. It is suspected that B cells act as antigen-presenting cells providing signals for clonal expansion and effector function of T cells. Activated B cells with RF specificity can be found in significant concentrations in the synovial membrane of patients with RA. B cells in RA synovium may function by secreting proinflammatory cytokines, such as IL-6, lymphotoxin, and TNF, that increase T-cell reactions leading to the pathology within synovium.

B cells and T cells interact to maintain bone homeostasis under normal conditions. B cells produce OPG; a member of the TNF receptor family that inhibits osteoclastogenesis,[16] and the production of OPG is regulated by T cell costimulation.[17] B cells account for greater than 60% of total OPG production in bone marrow. OPG blocks osteoclastogenesis by inhibiting the RANKL-RANK interaction by acting as a decoy receptor.[18] In vivo studies have shown that B-cell deficiency leads to significant reductions in OPG levels with increased bone resorption, whereas T-cell deficiency demonstrated reduced B-cell OPG secretion and increased bone loss.

Osteoblasts originate from pluripotent mesenchymal stem cells (MSC), which can also develop into adipocytes, chondrocytes, myoblasts, neurons, and tenocytes.[19] Bone-forming osteoblasts develop from progenitors through the activation of receptors expressed by MSC, such as bone morphogenetic proteins and the Wnt receptors' low-density lipoprotein receptor related proteins 5 and 6.[20] Osteoblasts produce high levels of Notch ligand jagged 1 and lead to an increase in MSC.[21] Through Notch activation, in vivo studies have demonstrated osteoblastic cells to be a regulatory component of the MSC niche that influences stem cell function.[22] Studies imply that inflammation within the arthritic bone impairs osteoblast ability to form sufficient mineralized bone. Osteoblasts express the cytokine RANKL and M-CSF, which are essential for osteoclast differentiation.[19] M-CSF is constitutively expressed by osteoblasts as opposed to the expression of RANKL, which is upregulated by factors such as parathyroid hormone and 1α, 25-dihydroxyvitamin D_3.[23] OC precursors bind to RANKL and differentiate into OCs in the presence of M-CSF.

Understanding the interaction between the immune and musculoskeletal systems in RA is essential. In addition to providing a basis for understanding the physiologic effects of synovectomy and periprosthetic osteolysis, it also provides an insight into the joint destructive process that leads to gait alteration and disability in the RA population.

GAIT ANALYSIS IN RA

Gait alteration secondary to the RA disease process should be understood, because it can affect procedure selection. Compared with HI, patients with RA walk with decreased speed, shorter step length, and longer stance phase at a preferred and fast self-selected speed.[24] Cadence and step width are not significantly different. When speed is normalized (0.8 m/s), and adjusted for weight, there is a significant difference in step length and cadence between patients with RA and HI. When velocity is controlled, patients with RA walk with shorter steps and increased cadence, whereas stance and step width are not significantly different between patients with RA and HI.

In patients with RA, cluster analyses reveal 3 specific gait strategies that are related to pathology rather than clinical severity level.[25] The first pattern is that patients with RA can demonstrate normal pressure through stance, with increased peak pressure at propulsion. This creates a wider contact area and limited ankle motion, which reduces peak pressures during propulsion. A second pattern demonstrates abnormal peak pressure curves with higher peak values specifically in propulsion phase. Forefoot deformity resulting in a stiffening of the foot-ankle complex is felt to create this pattern. A third pattern demonstrates an abnormal pressure pattern with significantly elevated peak pressures even in early stance. It is postulated that increased foot deformity with greater bony exposure reduces instantaneous contact areas leading to higher peak pressures in this pattern.

Although kinematic data for the hip and knee are lower in patients with RA than in HI, the most obvious difference is the reduced positive work at the ankle, which is the result of reduced plantar flexor moments during preswing.[26] This is thought to result from reduced walking speed, pain, and weakness in the posterior muscle group. Patients with RA demonstrate a decrease in joint motions, moments, and work in the lower limbs during gait as compared with HI.

The knee cannot be excluded during assessment of ankle pathology specific to the end-stage arthritis procedure selection. In patients with RA, knee motion decreases significantly in the sagittal plane.[27] Patients with severe inflammation without destruction show a limitation of sagittal plane motion in stance phase, whereas patients with knee joint destruction have shortened swing phase duration and decreased sagittal plane motion in swing phase.

In patients with RA, gait is affected differently when comparing AA with TAA. Piriou and colleagues[28] published the only study that directly compared gait between healthy controls and patients who have undergone either AA or TAA with a 3-component implant. The control, AA, and TAA groups each contained 12 patients. Data were obtained via 3-dimensional video and force plates with the patients walking barefoot. Neither intervention restored normal range of motion or walking speed. The AA group walked faster with a longer step length and an asymmetric gait than the TAA group. The AA group was accompanied by a far greater knee movement than the TAA and control groups. This compensation for absence of ankle motion may increase strain and lead to degenerative changes in patients with RA. TAA allowed for a stance phase that was closer to the control group in relation to ground reactive force and symmetry of timing. The TAA group had a significantly greater ankle range of motion than the AA group; however, it was still significantly less than the control group. It was not established if this movement in the TAA group was sufficient to preserve adjacent joints. Neither study group attained the speed of the control group. Patients with inflammatory arthritis were excluded from the study.

Regarding the effect of ankle or hindfoot arthrodesis on the kinematics (joint movements) and kinetics (forces involved in movement generation) of the hip and knee, patients with RA show a significant increase in hip extension and knee flexion range of motion after surgery.[29] A normalization of hip and knee moments is noted after fusion in patients with RA when compared with HI, which aids in forward progression. Work analysis that describes muscle action over time was also improved in the hip and knee after fusion. These improvements in work and joint moments in the hip and knee after fusion aid forward propulsion of the body and advancement of the swing leg.

Procedure selection for the patient with RA is not necessarily geared toward restoring a normal gait as found in HI but rather toward restoring a gait that is the highest functional level for each specific patient. The procedures chosen are targeted at reducing pain and improving functional capacity.

ANKLE JOINT SYNOVECTOMY

In the absence of significant damage assessed radiographically, synovectomy can be considered an appropriate treatment when medical management has not been successful in early-stage RA.[30] Even with the advent of biologic therapy, inflamed synovium can remain. An understanding of the physiologic process gives the surgeon an insight into the impact and potential effectiveness of ankle joint synovectomy in the patient with RA.

Chronic synovial hyperplasia facilitates most signs and symptoms in RA in addition to being a primary determinant in disease outcome. Angiogenesis in RA is imbalanced whereby perpetual new vessel formation occurs, enabling leukocyte transendothelial migration into the synovial tissue.[31] The substantial increase in cells, including fibroblast-like synoviocytes (FLS), is linked to the destruction of articular surfaces.[32] In vivo studies provide one explanation for pannus formation, it has been shown to result from RA-FLS inability to undergo apoptosis and through the secretion of soluble factors that prevent infiltrating B and T cells from undergoing programmed cell death.

Proliferation of the synovium precedes the cartilage destruction process.[33] It is presumed that RA synovium is involved in the induction of catabolic activities in joint cartilage. When stimulated, joint cartilage chondrocytes release matrix-degrading enzymes that lead to cartilage destruction.[33,34] Matrix metalloproteases (MMPs) 1, 3, 9, and 13 are such enzymes. Synovial fluid may be the transport vehicle for signaling molecules that regulate joint cartilage activity. Chemokines are soluble peptides that regulate cell movement, structure, development, and differentiation. Chemokine stromal cell–derived factor 1 (SDF-1) is derived from synovium and is increased more than 10 fold in patients with RA as compared with normal controls. The receptor for SDF-1, CXCR4 is expressed by chondrocytes and not by synovial fibroblasts. The interaction of SDF-1 and chondrocyte-expressed CXCR-4 propagates the release of MMP-3 by chondrocytes, leading to cartilage degradation in RA.

Synovectomy is effective in patients with RA because SDF-1 is removed by surgery preventing release of MMP-9 and MMP-13 from articular chondrocytes, preventing breakdown of cartilage.[35] Kanbe and colleagues[35] demonstrated in 28 patients with RA that SDF-1 was reduced 6.7 fold after arthroscopic synovectomy. Synovectomy can provide clinical long-term improvement. Pain reduction and increased joint mobility are more evident with minimal joint destruction on radiographs. Arthroscopic synovectomy is recommended for early intervention and open ankle synovectomy for late stage arthritis.[36]

Synovectomy does not provide a true joint-preserving effect. When compared with arthroscopic synovectomy in other RA joints, open synovectomy has traditionally been associated with loss of motion and longer rehabilitation time. Akagi and colleagues[37] assessed 20 ankles with RA that underwent arthroscopic synovectomy with an average follow-up of 15 years (range 10–25 years). The natural course of RA destruction was altered, and the anti-inflammatory effect of synovectomy was found to be long-standing.

Arthroscopic synovectomy is thought to enhance the efficacy of disease-modifying antirheumatic drug treatment. Open late ankle joint synovectomy allows for gains in ankle score due to pain reduction and increased mobility even though there may be a decline in function.[38] Anders and colleagues[38] demonstrated this in 29 patients with RA who underwent open ankle joint synovectomy. Synovectomy reduces symptoms but has not been found to prevent radiographic deterioration. Magnetic resonance imaging (MRI) can detect synovitis in early RA, which is highly predictive of future radiographic erosions.[39] Ostergaard and Ejberg[39] demonstrated a positive predictive value of 80% for erosive damage within 1 year of high synovial volumes and a negative predictive value of 100% in the presence of low synovial volume in patients with established RA.

Synovectomy in the absence of pain may be considered prophylactic; however, symptoms such as swelling and reduced function with MRI correlation may aid in diagnosing early synovitis. If appropriate medical management fails then synovectomy may delay the development of joint destruction. When synovectomy is no longer an option because of extensive joint destruction, AA and TAA should be considered.

ANKLE ARTHRODESIS

Performing AA requires an understanding of the effect of foot position during the procedure and its subsequent effect on gait. One of the earliest investigations for foot positioning in ankle fusion with gait analysis was performed by Mazur and colleagues.[40] Their observations provided a good foundation to build on in the field. They noted that some patients younger than 50 years could run after fusion, whereas no one older than 50 years was able to run. All patients developed marked calf atrophy with the muscles showing functional ability. This was suspected to lessen knee stability. Limb length discrepancy from fusion (0.3–1.3 cm) was rated as insignificant. Subtalar joint motion was significantly lessened, whereas midfoot motion substantially allowed dorsiflexion and plantar flexion. Radiographs revealed degenerative changes that did not correlate with symptoms. Increased plantar-flexed fusion position correlated with more severe degenerative changes. Gait analysis with shoes on showed minor alterations from normal controls. Preferred walking speed was decreased with cadence normal to slightly slower than HI. Step lengths of both the limbs in patients with fused ankles were symmetric and normal to controls. Single limb stance on the fused ankle was for a shorter duration than on the nonfused ankle. Adverse effects were more evident when walking barefoot. When the ankle was fused, midtarsal motion was the alternative to the combined foot and ankle motion in a normal subject. Fusing the subject in plantar flexion was found to cause genu recurvatum or toe walking. The absence of motion in smaller foot joints predisposed the patient to poorer results. An interesting conclusion from this study was that total ankle replacement should be considered in the presence of polyarticular small joint disease in the foot and the inability for these diseased joints to compensate for a fused ankle.

Other investigators have added to Mazur's work and further defined the optimum position for AA: neutral position of the ankle, about 5° of heel valgus, external rotation of the talus on the tibia (5°–10°) with posterior displacement of the talus on the tibia.[41] Buck and colleagues[42] showed that anterior translation of the talus on the tibia was associated with genu recurvatum during level walking. An internally positioned ankle fusion provides less sagittal plane motion of the hindfoot than neutral position provides. They emphasized the effect of fusion position with regard to how it could apply stress to the knee. AA has detrimental effects on the smaller joints of the foot and hence gait.[43] Combined sagittal plane motion decreases while the mean subtalar motion and mean medial column motion increases. This is a statistically significant relative hypermobility of the subtalar and medial column joints after ankle fusion. However, in the patient with RA these compensatory mechanisms may be lost because of joint destruction. This differed from Mazur's earlier findings of decreased subtalar joint motion.

Twenty-seven years after Mazur's study, Thomas and colleagues[44] published a gait analysis and functional outcomes study on 26 patients who underwent AA and compared them with 27 gender and age matched controls. They found that the study group had significant reductions in stride length and cadence than the controls. Gait velocity was also reduced. The positive effect of wearing shoes after surgery has not gone undocumented.[45] Walking in everyday shoes after fusion applies stress to the subtalar and midtarsal joints. Increasing the shoe instep delays heel-off and moves the ground reactive forces at heel-off closer to the metatarsal heads and away from the midfoot region. For patients whose ankles were fused in neutral position, it is recommended to consider shoes with a higher instep with the understanding that above a certain height level, it could alter knee dynamics or create a sense of instability. An optimum position has been defined for ankle fusion, whereas in patients who have fixed flexion deformities of the hip or knee that are not to be addressed, the fused position may need to be dorsiflexed beyond neutral to allow for an uncomplicated gait.

Gait studies have found an increase in force and peak pressures occurring in the talonavicular and calcaneocuboid joints after arthrodesis.[46,47] This may explain the increased degeneration that develops in the midfoot region. Ipsilateral arthritis of the smaller foot joints after AA is also a result of impaired biomechanics.[48] Most studies that reference this type of degeneration generally have not identified assessing preoperative radiographs for preexisting pathology. Sheridan and colleagues[48] reviewed preoperative and postoperative radiographs of 71 patients who underwent ankle fusion related to OA. They found that 68 (95.8%) sets of radiographs demonstrated preexisting arthritic changes in the midfoot and hindfoot. Patients with inflammatory arthritis were excluded from the study.

Biomechanical Properties of Fixation

Defining the best position for fusion depends on its ability to maintain near normal gait parameters with the least detrimental effects, whereas the ideal fixation for the patient with RA is dependent on bone quality. Numerous investigators have compared fixation methods for AA ranging from screw fixation, external fixation, various plating technologies, or a combination thereof.[49,50] Most of these studies include patients without RA or fail to account for bone quality. Over the last decade researchers have been using dual energy x-ray absorptiometry (DEXA) scan to define bone quality of cadaver specimens and bone models that better represent various degrees of bone density to compare fixation methods.[51] The biomechanical properties of specific bone composites have been validated to be comparable to human bone.[52]

A finite element analysis was performed by Alonso-Vázquez and colleagues[53] to test the effect of bone quality on the stability of AA by comparing 2-screw with 3-screw constructs in specimens of varying bone quality. They assessed the angle of screw insertion (30°, 45°, 60°, relative to long axis of tibia), origin of insertion and orientation of third screw (from anterior or posterior), level screws crossed fusion site (above, on, beneath), flat bone cuts versus maintaining morphology (intact cut), and bone quality. Three levels of bone quality were simulated: aged bone, osteoporotic bone, and highly osteoporotic bone. A reduced Young modulus of 10%, 33%, and 50% for the cortical bone and 26%, 66%, and 90% for the cancellous bone was used for the respective bone quality levels. Previous literary sources determined value reductions.[54,55]

Regardless of the number of screws, intact-cut arthrodesis was always associated with lower micromotion at the joint interface as compared with flat-cut arthrodesis. Screw insertion at 30° was always associated with the lowest micromotions regardless of the location of screw crossing or type of joint resection, that is, flat versus intact, or 2 versus 3 screws. Worsening of bone quality demonstrated a larger difference between screw configurations in 2-screw technique. The third screw when inserted in the anterior to posterior direction in poor quality bone allowed better stability in external torsion compared with a posterior to anterior insertion. It also provided better resistance against dorsiflexion in flat-cut arthrodesis. The posterior screw provided better resistance to dorsiflexion in intact arthrodesis. Overall, it was determined that intact joint preparation and 3-screw fixation with the medial and lateral screws inserted 30° to the long axis of the tibia provided the most stable construct in poor quality bone. This construct may not be good enough even in the worst quality bone. This study was supplemented by previous finite element analyses assessing 3-screw fixation for AA and flat cut versus intact joint contours for AA.[56,57] Screw orientation, screw insertion direction, and joint preparation were tested in these prior studies.

Previous biomechanical studies that compare crossed screws with parallel placed screws found that the crossed screw technique was more rigid especially in resisting torsional stresses.[58] Thordarson and colleagues[59] compared cancellous bone screws to a bilateral external fixation construct (Calandruccio triangular frame, Memphis, TN, USA). Although their findings were pertinent, it is the 5 cadaver specimens they excluded from their analyses that draw interest from a bone quality perspective. In these 5 specimens the bone quality and screw purchase was so poor that 4 N m of torque could not be sustained with screw fixation. Application of external fixation, with 4.5-mm threaded pins, afforded improved strength; however, large motion between the pins was noted, implying neither fixation method was satisfactory in a severely osteoporotic bone. They recommended that a mild torque be applied manually to the foot intraoperatively and if no motion is noted at the fusion site then the screws should be left in place. If motion is noted then screw removal with application of external fixation should be considered. Locking plates or intramedullary (IM) nail fixation may prove beneficial in osteopenic bone. Application of a fibular strut graft also improves torsional rigidity in bones of poor quality.[60] A biomechanical comparison of ring fixation and 3-screw fixation demonstrates no statistically significant differences in torsional stiffness, bending stiffness, or joint rotation under load.[61] When bone density is suboptimal or complex ankle pathology precludes screw fixation, external ring fixation is a viable option.

Concomitant symptomatic subtalar pathology in patients with RA is common, necessitating tibiotalocalcaneal (TTC) fusion. IM nails have demonstrated increased biomechanical stiffness in all bending and torsional directions.[62] Second generation angle–stable locking medullary nails and compressed angle–stable locking nails have demonstrated better stability than nails with static locking.[51] Breakage of the posterior-to-anterior calcaneal screw is a common failure pattern. Posterior-to-anterior calcaneal screw fixation demonstrates more stability than the lateral-to-medial screw orientation.[63] Augmenting medullary nails with a TTC screw improves stability of the fixation construct; typically, this screw is inserted from the posterior inferior calcaneus into the anterior tibia.[64] A benefit of medullary nail fixation is that it can be introduced percutaneously without the need for large incisions for application. Newer generation medullary nails when compared with multiplanar external fixation in biomechanical analysis on DEXA-assessed paired limbs have not demonstrated a significant difference in bending stiffness. Torsional stiffness has been found to be greater with ring fixation for arthrodesis.[65] Only a weak correlation was found between BMD and displacement.[66] Medullary nails and blade plates for TTC fusions have been compared with blade plates demonstrating reduced stability in torsion and inversion or eversion in the presence of low bone density.[67] Blade plates did demonstrate an increased initial stability in internal rotation. When a supplemental TTC screw is added to the blade plate construct, an increase in stability has been demonstrated and is superior to previous generation IM nails.[68] When compared biomechanically, locking plate fixation has provided better fixation in specimens with lower BMD than does blade plate fixation.[69] Fixation selection varies depending on the severity of the disease process. Ensuring that multiple fixation techniques are available at the time of surgery provides options when complications occur.

Numerous surgical approaches have been described for ankle fusion. Surgical techniques for the rheumatoid ankle are consistent with that of OA and posttraumatic arthritis. The choice of procedure is influenced by the presenting pathology, including severity of deformity, soft tissue envelope, and prior history, as well as the surgeon's familiarity with differing techniques. Before definitive treatment, evaluation of the more proximal extremity, including the knee, hip, and spine, must be performed, as well as identification of distal joint disease. Proximal joint disease should be addressed before ankle fusion. Subtalar pathology has been shown to precede ankle joint disease regularly in patients with RA and can alter procedure choice.[70] In addition to standard radiographic evaluation, computed tomographic (CT) examination allows for assessment of pathology within the osseous segments that may alter fixation choice (**Fig. 1**).

Open AA

The most common approach described for open ankle joint resection involves a lateral transfibular approach.[71] Regardless of the fixation method, fusion rates with the open technique have been acceptable. A fibular osteotomy approximately 4 cm proximal to the joint line provides access to the tibiotalar joint surfaces. The posterior fibular soft tissue attachments may be left intact. Resection of the medial joint gutter is more readily afforded by a separate medial incision, although tilting of the talus and use of curved hand instrumentation can facilitate medial gutter debridement through a transfibular approach. A complete resection of the medial malleolus is optional; however, leaving the malleoli increases rotational stability. Joint resection can maintain the joint morphology or entail flat cuts. When varus deformity is present lateral bone resection is performed. When valgus deformity is present medial bone is resected. In the presence of severe frontal plane ankle joint deformity or bone loss, TTC fusion may be considered. Use of the fibula as an onlay graft or as a graft within the fusion site is at the discretion of the surgeon. Preparation of the fibula as an onlay graft requires decorticating the medial aspect with resection of the articular cartilage. The lateral aspect of the tibia can be fish-scaled to promote fusion to the onlay graft. Internal and external fixations have demonstrated acceptable fusion rates.

A review of 32 open ankle arthrodeses by Cracchiolo and colleagues[72] in patients with RA demonstrated that fusion occurred in 15 out of 19 (79%) patients fixated with external fixation and 10 out of 13 (77%) patients fixated with internal fixation. Four externally fixated patients and 1 internally fixated patient developed infections. The method of fixation did not affect the time of healing. Four of the seven failed fusions were taking an average of 17 mg of prednisone daily. In 11 of the 19 fusions, patients were taking an average of 6 mg daily. Miehlke and colleagues[73] described a lateral transfibular approach with internal screw fixation that demonstrated a 92% fusion rate at 16 weeks in 43 patients; 41 had RA. Two ankle nonunions and 2 infections occurred in patients who underwent pantalar fusion. A separate study by

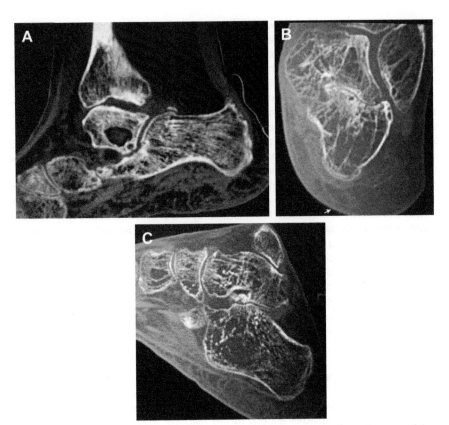

Fig. 1. (*A, B, C*) CT images of different patients demonstrating various degrees of bone quality.

Dereymaeker and colleagues[74] reviewed 14 open AA in patients with RA. Ten were fixated with external fixation, 3 with cannulated screws, and one by fibular strut graft with a short walking cast. Six of the ten externally fixated patients had a fibular strut graft. Five nonunions occurred, 1 from those with a fibular strut graft and 4 from those without the graft. No infections were encountered and only 1 delayed wound healing occurred. The strut graft was inserted into the talus and the tibia impacted onto it similar to an IM nail concept. They concluded that the addition of the fibular strut graft improved healing in the rheumatoid population. Felix and Kitaoka[75] reviewed 26 ankles in patients with RA, 14 tibiotalar fusions, and 12 TTC fusions. Twenty patients had external fixation and 6 patients had 3-screw fixation with fibular onlay graft. Twenty-five of twenty-six (96%) ankles fused without any infections. Two patients experienced delayed wound healing. In patients with RA, a single technique for AA achieved 18/20 (90%) fusion rate as described by Kennedy and colleagues.[76] An open technique with fibular osteotomy using the fibula as an onlay graft with the medial malleolus resected and 3 parallel screws for fixation was performed. There were 2 superficial and 1 deep infection. The lateral approach provides reproducible and predictable results in the RA population. However, not all patients are candidates for this approach, and the surgeon needs to be familiar with alternate techniques.

A medial joint approach is an option that may prove beneficial when there is concern for wound healing complications involving the lateral soft tissue envelope. In the presence of severe valgus deformity, corrective surgery with realignment can apply significant tension to the lateral side leading to wound complications (**Fig. 2**). This medial incision can be extended to allow for a single incision to incorporate triple arthrodesis.[77] Schuberth and colleagues[78] described a medial approach for AA in 13 patients. The medial malleolus was transected maintaining its attachment to the deltoid ligament. Fibular osteotomy when needed was typically performed through the medial incision. They had a 92% (12/13) fusion rate. Mann and colleagues[79] performed a medial approach for ankle fusion with a dowel technique in 7 patients with end-stage arthritis from hemophilia A and 1 patient with hemophilia B. The dowel was rotated 90° and the site held with compression staples. Fusion was achieved in 7 patients by 12 weeks and in 1 patient at 16 weeks. Care must be taken with medial joint approach because open plating techniques of the medial tibia have demonstrated significant compromise to the extra osseous blood supply of the metaphyseal region as compared with percutaneous techniques.[80] Further concern is that considerable arterial supply for the talus comes from the medial aspect, from the posterior tibial artery via the artery of the tarsal canal and deltoid branches.[81] Regardless of the fixation used or incision approach with the open technique, fusion rates have been acceptable in the rheumatoid population.

Arthroscopic AA

The arthroscopic approach is for end-stage joint disease without significant deformity.[82] A standard 2-portal approach is recommended. A third portal for outflow can improve visualization. Distraction of the joint can be obtained via a noninvasive distracter or external fixator. After synovectomy the articular cartilage is removed

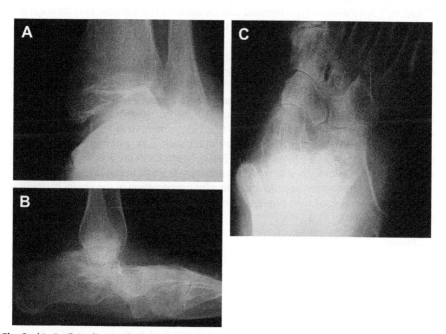

Fig. 2. (*A, B, C*) Radiographs demonstrating valgus deformity in rheumatoid ankle and foot. Due to the severity of deformity, lateral skin placement may undergo excessive tension after surgical reduction, leading to wound complications. Medial approach may prove advantageous in certain cases.

with burs and curettes. Fluoroscopy guides percutaneous screw insertion. This technique requires significant familiarity with arthroscopy. Care must be taken to prevent thermal necrosis of the bone from overzealous resection with the bur as this may complicate bone healing. The arthroscopic approach may prove beneficial in the presence of a compromised soft tissue envelope. External fixation and IM nailing are not precluded with this approach.

Nielsen and colleagues[83] compared 58 arthroscopy-guided ankle arthrodeses (6 patients with RA) with 49 open arthrodeses (2 patients with RA). The open technique group had the fibula and a portion of the tibia resected. The fusion site was fixated with 2 screws directed medially from the lateral talus angled approximately 45° to the long axis of the tibia. The arthroscopic fixation involved 2 screws inserted from the medial tibia into the talus angled 45° from the long axis of the tibia. Union rate at 1 year was 95% in the arthroscopy group and 84% in the open group. Twelve weeks after surgery, 90% of the arthroscopy and 57% of the open group showed bony union. The arthroscopy group was discharged on an average of 2.27 days earlier. They recommended that arthroscopy not be considered for varus or valgus deformities greater than 5°. Turan and colleagues[84] achieved a 100% fusion rate in 10 RA ankle fusion procedures through an arthroscopic technique. The mean time to fusion was 10 weeks (range 6–12 weeks) with no complications. Six procedures had simultaneous subtalar fusion (technique not described) and all ankles were fused via 2 crossed screws. Turan's study had similar results to that of Ogilve-Harris and colleagues[85] that obtained 17/19 (89%) rate of fusion in OA ankles. Ten ankles were fused by 8 weeks, 5 ankles by 12 weeks, and 2 by the sixth month after surgery. Two screws from the tibia and 1 from the fibula fixated the ankle joint. No postoperative infections were encountered. Incorporation of arthroscopic joint preparation with IM nailing for patients with RA has also been described for TTC fusion.[86] A mini–open type method can be used for the subtalar joint through a 1-cm incision with joint preparation via curettage.

Mini–Arthrotomy Arthrodesis Technique

Like the arthroscopic approach the mini-open or mini-arthrotomy technique is reserved for joints with minimal deformity.[87] Two small incisions, about 2 cm in length, are created medially and laterally in the approximate area of the standard arthroscopic portals. Baby lamina spreaders and external distractors can provide greater visualization. Joint debridement is performed with hand instrumentation such as osteotomes and curettes. Internal fixation is guided by fluoroscopy, or external fixation can be applied if internal fixation is not adequate. The concern for thermal necrosis is avoided with this technique, although still minimally affecting the soft tissue envelope. Both the arthroscopic and mini-open procedures allow for preservation of the fibula. In younger patients these techniques may prove advantageous if later in life they elect to have the arthrodesis converted to a TAA.

Percutaneous Technique

A less studied approach is the percutaneous technique that is performed when alignment is satisfactory.[88–90] Three different studies involved a total of 49 patients with RA who underwent percutaneous screw fixation without any joint debridement. Fusion occurred successfully in 45 of 49 (92%) patients. It was assumed as a result of the progressive joint destructive process that even when some cartilage remains over time with stable fixation, autofusion occurs as a result of autoimmune destruction of remaining cartilage.

When the soft tissue envelope precludes a more traditional approach, access to the ankle and subtalar joints can be obtained through a posterior approach. Hansen and

Cracchiolo[91] described a posterior approach with blade plate for TTC fusion in 10 patients in which fusion occurred successfully in all patients at a mean time of 14.5 weeks. There was 1 wound healing complication and 3 patients required plate removal due to pain. An anterior approach for ankle fusion has been described and is more typical during conversion of failed TAAs to AA as this incision placement is required for component removal.[92] Ankle fusion, when successful, provides acceptable outcomes. Although radiographic fusion can be demonstrated on plain radiographs, CT examination provides a more definitive assessment that may better determine bony consolidation. AA is an appropriate choice in RA cases associated with severe bone loss, neuropathy, and paralysis regardless of patient age.

AA VERSUS TAA

Comparison studies provide a unique assessment of TAA and AA outcomes from within the same surgical groups or centers. Four such studies including 1 meta-analysis are provided. McGuire and colleagues[93] reviewed outcomes that compared TAA with AA.[94] TAA was performed in 25 ankles with 10 RA ankles in the group. Eighteen patients underwent AA. The follow-up averaged 3.8 years with an average age of 49.5 years. Fusion in the arthrodesis group was done using a Charley compression technique (11 patients) with interposed iliac bone graft (7 patients). There was no mention of patients with RA in this group. Posttraumatic arthrosis (14 patients), failed ankle arthroplasty (3 patients), and postinfectious arthritis (1 patient) were the indications for AA. The average age was 41.3 years with an average follow-up of 3.3 years. The arthrodesis group (18 patients) had 14 (77%) excellent, 3 (16%) good, 0 fair, 0 poor, and 1 (6%) failed results. The arthroplasty group (25 patients) had 9 (36%) excellent, 9 (36%) good, 0 fair, 2 poor, and 5 (20%) failed results. Koefoed and Stürup[94] performed a prospective study comparing 14 ankle arthrodeses with 14 TAAs. The average age was 54 years (range 27–71 years) and 39 years (range 21–68 years) for the TAA and AA groups respectively. The average age for the arthritis subset groups was 48 years (range 45–50 years) and 24 years (21–31 years) for the TAA and AA groups. Four ankles in each group had RA. All surgeries were performed between 1981 and 1985. Median follow-up was 84 months. Arthrodeses were performed with a Charnley frame and arthroplasty was performed with a 2-piece cemented implant. The AA group had 4 deep infections, 3 nonunions, and development of subtalar arthrosis in 5 patients. The TAA group had no deep infections, 3 cases of skin necrosis, 1 revisional arthrodesis, and no development of subtalar arthrosis. They found that the arthroplasty group had better pain relief, function, and lower infection rate without the development of subtalar arthritis.

Soohoo and colleagues[95] compared reoperation rates between 4705 ankle arthrodeses and 480 ankle replacements during a 10-year study period (1995–2004). Six percent of the ankle fusion patients and 10% of the TAA patients had RA. Rates of revision surgery were 9% at 1 year and 23% at 5 years in the TAA group. Corresponding rates of revision in the arthrodesis group were 5% and 11%. Patients who had an AA had a 2.8% occurrence of subtalar fusion at 5 years as compared with TAA rate of 0.7%. Regression analysis confirmed a significant increase in the risk of major revision surgery in the TAA group.

Saltzman and colleagues[96] performed a nonrandomized study with concurrent controls as part of the study by Food and Drug Administration to evaluate the safety and efficacy of the Scandanavian Total Ankle Replacement (STAR) implant to treat arthritis. The pivotal STAR group included 158 ankles and the pivotal fusion group included 66 ankles. A continued access STAR group (N = 435) was also evaluated.

Patients with RA accounted for 12.7% of the STAR group and 6.5% of the fusion group. The pivotal groups were similar in gender, race, height, and weight. With the exception of pain, and an expected loss of motion in the fusion group, operative site adverse events were higher in the STAR pivotal group. These events included nerve injury, bone fracture, edema, wound problems, and bony changes. With the exception of infection major complications were also higher in the STAR group. The STAR group performed better in most functional scoring subscales except for pain relief, walking, and the presence of a limp.

Haddad and colleagues[97] compared 852 TAAs with 1262 ankle arthrodeses in a systematic review of the literature. Between 1990 and 1997, 56% of the arthrodesis studies were published, and all of the TAA studies were published between 1998 and 2005. Follow-up was from 2 to 9 years for the TAA group and 2 to 23 years for the arthrodesis group. Results in the TAA group were 38% excellent, 30.5% good, 5.5% fair, and 24% poor with a 7% revision rate. The survival rates after 5 and 10 years were 78% and 77% respectively. The corresponding results in the arthrodesis group were 31%, 37%, 13%, and 13% with a 9% revision rate. The main reason for revision was nonunion (65%).

SUMMARY

Synovectomy, AA, and TAA each have distinctive roles in the rheumatoid ankle. As a better understanding of the rheumatoid disease process occurs, targeted therapy may reduce or suppress progressive destruction, leading to improved outcomes regardless of the procedure chosen. Each procedure presents with its own unique complications and must be balanced against the patient's functional requirements and physiologic status. The surgeon needs to assess each patient individually relying on their experience and the use of the current and best evidence.

REFERENCES

1. Schett G. Osteoimmunology in rheumatic diseases. Arthritis Res Ther 2009;11: 210.
2. McInnes I, Schett G. Cytokines in the pathogenesis of rheumatoid arthritis. Nat Immunol 2007;7:429–42.
3. Bromley M, Wooley DE. Chondroclasts and osteoclasts at subchondral sites of erosion in the rheumatoid joint. Arthritis Rheum 1984;27:968–75.
4. Teitlebaum SL. Osteoclasts: what do they do and how do they do it? Am J Pathol 2007;170:427–35.
5. Takayanagi H, Oda H, Yamamoto S, et al. A new mechanism of bone destruction in rheumatoid arthritis: synovial fibroblasts induce osteoclastogenesis. Biochem Biophys Res Commun 1997;240:279–86.
6. Sato K, Takayanagi H. Osteoclasts, rheumatoid arthritis, and osteoimmunology. Curr Opin Rheumatol 2006;18:419–26.
7. Gravallese EM, Manning C, Tsay A, et al. Synovial tissue in rheumatoid arthritis is a source of osteoclast differentiation factor. Arhtritis Rheum 2000;43(2):250–8.
8. Kong YY, Yoshida H, Sarosi I, et al. OPGL is a key regulator of osteoclastogenesis, lymphocyte development and lymph node organogenesis. Nature 1999;397: 315–23.
9. Hofbauer LC, Lacey DL, Dunstan CR, et al. Interleukin-1β and tumor necrosis factor-α, but not interleukin-6, stimulate osteoprotegerin ligand gene expression in human osteoblastic cells. Bone 1999;25:255–9.

10. Lam J, Takeshita S, Barker E, et al. TNF-α induces osteoclastogenesis by direct stimulation of macrophages exposed to permissive levels of RANK ligand. J Clin Invest 2000;106:1481–8.
11. Wong BR, Josien R, Choi Y. TRANCE is a TNF family member that regulates dendritic cell and osteoclast function. J Leukoc Biol 1999;65:715–24.
12. Tagayanagi H, Ogasawara K, Hida S, et al. T-cell mediated regulation of osteo-clastogenesis by signaling cross-talk between RANKL and IFN-γ. Nature 2000; 408:600–5.
13. Kong YY, Feige U, Sarosi I, et al. Activated T-cells regulate bone loss and joint destruction in adjuvant arthritis through osteoprotegerin ligand. Nature 1999; 402:304–9.
14. Ouyang W, Kolls JK, Zheng Y. The biological functions of T-helper 17 cell effector cytokines in inflammation. Immunity 2008;28:454–67.
15. Kotake S, Udagawa N, Takahashi N, et al. IL-17 in synovial fluids from patients with rheumatoid arthritis is a potent stimulator of osteoclastogenesis. J Clin Invest 1999;103:1345–52.
16. Li Y, Toraido G, Li A, et al. B cells and T cells are critical for the preservation of bone homeostasis and attainment of peak bone mass in vivo. Blood 2007;109: 3838–49.
17. Lacey DL, Timms E, Tan HL, et al. Osteoprotegerin ligand is a cytokine that regu-lates osteoclast differentiation and activation. Cell 1998;93:165–76.
18. Gortz B, Hayer S, Redlich K. Arthritis induces lymphocytic bone marrow inflam-mation and endosteal bone formation. J Bone Miner Res 2004;19:990–8.
19. Yamamoto Y, Udagawa N, Matsuura S, et al. Osteoblasts provide a suitable microenvironment for the action of receptor activator of nuclear factor-kappaB ligand. Endocrinology 2006;147(7):3366–74.
20. Walsh MC, Kim N, Kadono Y, et al. Osteoimmunology, interplay between the immune system and bone metabolism. Annu Rev Immunol 2006;24:33–63.
21. Yamaguchi A, Kamori T, Suda T. Regulation of osteoblast differentiation modu-lated by bone morphogenetic proteins, hedgehogs and Cbfa1. Endocr Rev 2000;21:393–411.
22. Mensah K, Schwarz E. The emerging field of osteoimmunology. Immunol Res 2009;45(2–3):100–13.
23. Calvi LM, Sims NA, Hunzelman JL, et al. Activated parathyroid hormone/parathy-roid hormone related protein receptor in osteoblastic cells differentially affects cortical and trabecular bone. J Clin Invest 2001;107:277–86.
24. Eppeland S, Mykelbust G, Hodt-Billington C, et al. Gait patterns in subjects with rheumatoid arthritis cannot be explained by reduced speed alone. Gait Posture 2009;29:499–503.
25. Giacomozzi C, Martelli F, Nagel A, et al. Cluster analysis to classify gait alterations in rheumatoid arthritis using peak pressure curves. Gait Posture 2009;29:220–4.
26. Weiss R, Wretenberg P, Stark A, et al. Gait pattern in rheumatoid arthritis. Gait Posture 2008;28:229–34.
27. Sakauchi M, Narushima K, Sone H, et al. Kinematic approach to gait analysis in patients with rheumatoid arthritis involving the knee joint. Arthritis Rheum 2001; 45:35–41.
28. Piriou P, Culpan P, Mullins M, et al. Ankle replacement versus arthrodesis: a comparative gait analysis study. Foot Ankle Int 2008;29(1):3–9.
29. Weiss R, Brostrom E, Stark A, et al. Ankle/hindfoot arthrodesis in rheumatoid arthritis improves kinematics and kinetics of the knee and hip: a prospective gait analysis study. Rheumatology 2007;46:1024–8.

30. American college of rheumatology subcommittee on rheumatoid arthritis guidelines. Guidelines for the management of rheumatoid arthritis 2002 update. Arthritis Rheum 2002;46(2):328–46.
31. Szekanecz Z, Koch A. Angiogenesis and its targeting in rheumatoid arthritis. Vascul Pharmacol 2009;51(1):1–7.
32. Korb A, Pavenstadt H. Cell death in rheumatoid arthritis. Apoptosis 2009;14: 447–54.
33. Kanbe K, Takagishi K, Chen Q. Stimulation of matrix metalloproteases 3 release from human chondrocytes by the interaction of stromal cell-derived factor-1 and cxc Chemokine receptor 4. Arthritis Rheum 2002;46(1):130–2.
34. Chiu Y, Yang R, Hsieh K, et al. Stromal cell-derived factor -1 induces matrix metalloproteases-13 expression in human chondrocytes. Mol Pharmacol 2007;72: 695–703.
35. Kanbe K, Takemura T, Takeuchi K, et al. Synovectomy reduces stromal-cell-derived factor-1 (sdf-1) which is involved in the destruction of cartilage in osteoarthritis and rheumatoid arthritis. J Bone Joint Surg Br 2004;86(2):296–300.
36. Carl H, Swoboda B. [Effectiveness of arthroscopic synovectomy in rheumatoid arthritis]. Z Rheumatol 2008;67(6):485–90 [in German].
37. Akagi S, Sugano H, Ogawa R. The long-term results of ankle joint synovectomy for rheumatoid arthritis. Clin Rheumatol 1997;16(3):284–90.
38. Anders S, Schaumburger J, Kerl S, et al. [Long-term results of synovectomy in the rheumatoid ankle joint]. Z Rheumatol 2007;66(7):595–602 [in German].
39. Ostergard M, Ejberg B. Magnetic resonance imaging of the synovium in rheumatoid arthritis. Semin Musculoskelet Radiol 2004;8(4):287–99.
40. Mazur J, Schwartz E, Simon S. Ankle arthrodesis. Long-term follow-up with gait analysis. J Bone Joint Surg Am 1979;61(7):964–75.
41. Thomas R, Daniels T. Current concepts review. Ankle arthritis. J Bone Joint Surg Am 2003;85(5):923–36.
42. Buck P, Morrey B, Chao E. The optimum position of arthrodesis of the ankle. A gait study of the knee and ankle. J Bone Joint Surg Am 1987;69:1052–62.
43. Sealey RJ, Myerson MS, Molloy A, et al. Sagittal plane motion of the hindfoot following ankle arthrodesis: a prospective analysis. Foot Ankle Int 2009;30(3): 187–96.
44. Thomas R, Daniels T, Parker K. Gait analysis and functional outcomes following ankle arthrodesis for isolated ankle arthritis. J Bone Joint Surg Am 2006;88(3): 526–34.
45. Beyaert C, Sirveaux F, Paysant J, et al. The effect of tibio-talar arthrodesis on foot kinematics and ground reaction force progression during walking. Gait Posture 2004;20:84–91.
46. Jung HG, Parks BG, Nguyen A, et al. Effect of tibiotalar joint arthrodesis on adjacent tarsal joint pressure in a cadaver model. Foot Ankle Int 2007;28(1): 103–8.
47. Suckel A, Muller O, Herberts T, et al. Changes in chopart joint load following tibiotalar arthrodesis: in vitro analysis of 8 cadaver specimen in a dynamic model. BMC Musculoskelet Disord 2007;8:80.
48. Sheridan B, Robinson D, Hubble M, et al. Ankle arthrodesis and its relationship to Ipsilateral arthritis of the hind- and mid-foot. J Bone Joint Surg Br 2006;88:206–7.
49. Nasson S, Shuff C, Palmer D, et al. Biomechanical comparison of ankle arthrodesis techniques: crossed screws vs. blade plate. Foot Ankle Int 2001;22(7): 575–80.

50. Mueckley T, Eichorn S, von Oldenberg G, et al. Biomechanical evaluation of primary stiffness of tibiotalar arthrodesis with an Intramedullary compression nail and four other fixation devices. Foot Ankle Int 2006;27(10):814–20.
51. Muckley T, Hoffmeir K, Klos K, et al. Angle-stable and compressed angle-stable locking for tibiotalocalcaneal arthrodesis with retrograde intramedullary nails. J Bone Joint Surg Am 2008;90(3):620–7.
52. Cristogolini L, Viceconti M. Mechanical validation of whole bone composite tibia models. J Biomech 2000;29:525–35.
53. Alonso-Vázquez A, Lauge-Pedersen L, Lidgren L, et al. The effect of bone quality on the stability of ankle arthrodesis. A finite element study. Foot Ankle Int 2004; 25(11):840–50.
54. Ding M, Dalstra M, Danielson C, et al. Age variations in the properties of human tibial trabecular bone. J Bone Joint Surg Br 1997;79:995–1002.
55. Zioupos P, Currey J. Changes in the stiffness, strength and toughness of human cortical bone with age. Bone 1998;22:57–66.
56. Alonso-Vazquez A, Lauge-Pederson H, Lidgren L, et al. Initial stability of ankle arthrodesis with three-screw fixation. A finite element analysis. Clin Biomech 2004;19:751–9.
57. Alonso-Vazquez A, Lauge-Pederson H, Lidgren L, et al. Finite element analysis of the initial stability of ankle arthrodesis with internal; fixation: flat cut versus intact joint contours. Clin Biomech 2003;18:244–53.
58. Friedman RL, Glisson RR, Nunley JA. A biomechanical comparative analysis of two techniques for tibiotalar arthrodesis. Foot Ankle Int 1994;15(6):301–5.
59. Thordarson D, Markolf K, Cracchiolo A. Stability of an ankle arthrodesis fixed by cancellous bone-screws compared with that fixed by an external fixator. A biomechanical study. J Bone Joint Surg Am 1992;74(7):1050–5.
60. Thordarson D, Mrkolf K, Cracchiolo A. Arthrodesis of the ankle with cancellous-bone screws and fibular strut graft. Biomechanical analysis. J Bone Joint Surg Am 1990;72(9):1359–63.
61. Ogut T, Glisson R, Chuckpaiwong B, et al. External ring fixation versus screw fixation for ankle arthrodesis: a biomechanical comparison. Foot Ankle Int 2009; 30(4):353–60.
62. Berend ME, Glisson RR, Nunley JA. A biomechanical comparison of Intramedullary nail and crossed lag screw fixation for tibiotalocalcaneal arthrodesis. Foot Ankle Int 1997;18(10):639–43.
63. Means KR, Parks BG, Nuyen A, et al. Intramedullary nail fixation with posterior-to-anterior compared to transverse distal screw placement for tibiotalocalcaneal arthrodesis: a biomechanical investigation. Foot Ankle Int 2006;27(12): 1137–42.
64. O'neill PJ, Parks BG, Walsh R, et al. Biomechanical analysis of screw-augmented intramedullary fixation for tibiotalocalcaneal arthrodesis. Foot Ankle Int 2007; 28(7):804–9.
65. Santangelo JR, Glisson RR, Garras DN, et al. Tibiotalocalcaneal arthrodesis: a biomechanical comparison of multiplanar external fixation with intramedullary fixation. Foot Ankle Int 2008;29(9):936–41.
66. Fragomen AT, Meyers KN, Davis N, et al. A biomechanical comparison of micromotion after ankle fusion using 2 fixation techniques: Intramedullary arthrodesis nail or ilizarov external fixator. Foot Ankle Int 2008;29(3):334–41.
67. Alfahd U, Roth S, Stephen D, et al. Biomechanical comparison of intramedullary nail and blade plate fixation for tibiotalocalcaneal arthrodesis. J Orthop Trauma 2005;19(10):703–8.

68. Chiodo C, Acevedo J, Sammarco J, et al. Intramedullary rod fixation compared with blade- plate-and- screw fixation for tibiotalocalcaneal arthrodesis: a biomechanical investigation. J Bone Joint Surg Am 2003;85(12):2425–8.

69. Chiodos MD, Parks BG, Schon, et al. Blade plate compared with locking plate for tibiotalocalcaneal arthrodesis: a cadaver study. Foot Ankle Int 2008;29(2): 219–24.

70. Belt E, Kaarela K, Maenpaa H, et al. Relationship of ankle joint involvement with subtalar destruction in patients with rheumatoid arthritis. A 20-year follow-up study. J Bone Joint Surg 2001;68:154–7.

71. Es Holt, Hansen ST, Mayo KA, et al. Ankle arthrodesis using internal screw fixation. Clin Orthop Relat Res 1991;268:21–7.

72. Cracchiolo A, Cimino W, Lian G. Arthrodesis of the ankle in patients who have rheumatoid arthritis. J Bone Joint Surg Am 1992;74(6):903–9.

73. Miehlke W, Gschwend N, Rippstein P, et al. Compression arthrodesis of the rheumatoid ankle and hindfoot. Clin Orhtop Relat Res 1997;340:75–86.

74. Dereymaeker G, Van Eygen P, Driesen, et al. Tibiotalar arthrodesis in the rheumatoid foot. Clin Orthop Relat Res 1998;349:43–7.

75. Felix N, Kitaoka H. Ankle arthrodesis in patients with rheumatoid arthritis. Clin Orthop 1998;349:58–64.

76. Kennedy J, Harty J, Casey K, et al. Outcome after single technique ankle arthrodesis in patients with rheumatoid arthritis. Clin Orthop Relat Res 2003;412:131–8.

77. Jeng C, Vora A, Myerson M. The medial approach to triple arthrodesis. Indications and technique for management of rigid valgus deformities in high-risk patients. Foot Ankle Clin 2005;10:515–21.

78. Schuberth J, Cheung C, Rush S, et al. The medial approach for arthrodesis of the ankle: a report of 13 cases. J Foot Ankle Surg 2005;44(2):125–32.

79. Mann H, Biring G, Choudhury M, et al. Ankle arthropathy in the haemophilic patient: a description of a novel ankle arthrodesis technique. Haemophilia 2009;15:458–63.

80. Borrelli J, Prickett W, Song E, et al. Extraosseous blood supply of the tibia and the effects of different plating techniques: a human cadaveric study. J Orthop Trauma 2002;16(10):691–5.

81. Giebel G, Meyer C, Koebke J, et al. The arterial supply of the ankle joint and its importance for the operative fracture treatment. Surg Radiol Anat 1997;19: 231–5.

82. Myerson MS, Quill G. Ankle arthrodesis; a comparison of an arthroscopic and an open method of treatment. Clin Orthop Relat Res 1991;20:368–74.

83. Nielsen K, Linde F, Jensen N. The outcome of arthroscopic and open surgery ankle arthrodesis. A comparative retrospective study of 107 patients. Foot Ankle Surg 2008;14:153–7.

84. Turan I, Wredmark T, Fellander-Tsai L. Arthroscopic ankle arthrodesis in rheumatoid arthritis. Clin Orthop Relat Res 1995;320:110–4.

85. Ogilve-Harris D, Lieberman I, Fitsialos D. Arthroscopically assisted arthrodesis for osteoarthritic ankles. J Bone Joint Surg Am 1993;75(8):1167–74.

86. Sekiya H, Horii T, Kariya Y, et al. Arthroscopic-assisted tibiotalocalcaneal arthrodesis using intramedullary nail with fins: a case report. J Foot Ankle Surg 2006; 45(4):266–70.

87. Paremain GD, Miller SD, Myerson MS. Ankle arthrodesis: results after the mini arthrotomy technique. Foot Ankle Int 1996;17:247–52.

88. Lauge-Pedersen H, Knutson K, Rydholm U. Percutaneous ankle arthrodesis in the rheumatoid patient without debridement of the joint. Foot 1998;8:226–9.

89. Lauge-Pedersen H. Percutaneous arthrodesis. Acta Orthop Scand 2003;74(307): 1–30.
90. Anderson T, Maxander P, Rydholm U, et al. Ankle arthrodesis by compression screws in rheumatoid arthritis. Acta Orthop 2005;76(6):884–90.
91. Hanson TW, Cracchiolo A. The use of 95 degree blade plate and a posterior approach to achieve tibiotalocalcaneal arthrodesis. Foot Ankle Int 2002;23(8): 704–10.
92. Culpan P, Le Strat V, Piriou P, et al. Arthrodesis after failed total ankle replacement. J Bone Joint Surg Br 2007;89:1178–83.
93. McGuire M, Kyle R, Gustilo R, et al. Comparative analysis of ankle arthroplasty versus ankle arthrodesis. Clin Orthop Relat Res 1988;226:174–81.
94. Koefoed H, Stürup J. Comparison of ankle arthroplasty and arthrodesis. A prospective series with long term follow-up. Foot 1994;4:6–9.
95. SooHoo N, Zingmond D, Ko C. Comparison of reoperation rates following ankle arthrodesis and total ankle arthroplasty. J Bone Joint Surg 2007;89:2143–9.
96. Saltzman C, Mann R, Ahrens J, et al. Prospective controlled trial of STAR total ankle replacement versus ankle fusion: initial results. Foot Ankle Int 2009;30(7): 579–93.
97. Haddad S, Coetzee J, Estok R, et al. Intermediate and long-term outcomes of total ankle arthroplasty and ankle arthrodesis. J Bone Joint Surg 2007;89: 1899–905.

Total Ankle Arthroplasty in the Rheumatoid Patient

Lawrence A. DiDomenico, DPM[a,b,c,*], Joseph R. Treadwell, DPM[d], Laurence Z. Cain, DPM[b]

KEYWORDS

• Rheumatoid arthritis • Total ankle arthroplasty
• Total ankle replacement • Rheumatoid disease
• Ankle arthrodesis

Rheumatoid arthritis is a systemic disease that commonly affects the foot and ankle joints. It is an autoimmune connective tissue disorder that specifically targets synovial membranes, thus causing inflammatory arthritis.[1] As the disease progresses, adjacent cartilage and bone erode, leading to joint destruction. There is a connection. Evidence has shown a clear pattern of hindfoot involvement following rheumatoid arthritis diagnosis.[2] The most common finding is ankle valgus (varus deformities are rare), which is reported as high as 29% among those who had rheumatoid arthritis disease for more than 5 years. Reports also indicate that the tibiotalar joint is affected in up to 50% of rheumatic patients.[3] Furthermore, in correlation to clinical findings, one study has demonstrated that nearly half of patients who have had the disease for more than 13 years report hindfoot symptoms worse than forefoot symptoms.[4]

A myriad of surgical procedures are available for treatment of the rheumatoid forefoot. These include arthrodesis, total joint implants, hemi-joint implants, joint resection, and joint-sparing techniques.[5] In sharp contrast, however, procedures for the hindfoot are limited to total ankle replacement and arthrodesis. Joint fusion has long endured as the gold standard for treatment. Unfortunately fusion imparts stress on adjacent joints, leading to further joint destruction and subsequent intervention. Ankle arthroplasty provides a feasible option.

[a] Ohio College of Podiatric Medicine, Youngstown, OH, USA
[b] Reconstructive Rearfoot & Ankle Surgical Fellowship, Ankle and Foot Care Centers/Ohio College of Podiatric Medicine, 8175 Market Street, Youngstown, OH, USA
[c] Section of Podiatric Medicine and Surgery, St Elizabeth's Medical Center, Youngstown, OH, USA
[d] Foot & Ankle Specialists of Connecticut, PC, 6 Germantown Road, Danbury, CT 06810, USA
* Corresponding author. Reconstructive Rearfoot & Ankle Surgical Fellowship, Ankle and Foot Care Centers/Ohio College of Podiatric Medicine, 8175 Market Street, Youngstown, OH.
E-mail address: LD5353@aol.com

Clin Podiatr Med Surg 27 (2010) 295–311
doi:10.1016/j.cpm.2010.01.001
0891-8422/10/$ – see front matter © 2010 Elsevier Inc. All rights reserved.

podiatric.theclinics.com

BACKGROUND

Total ankle arthroplasty (TAA) allows motion and reduces stresses on proximal and distal joints as compared with ankle arthrodesis.[6] A proper review of the literature about TAA in patients with rheumatoid arthritis requires a basic appreciation of the progression of implant design as well as an understanding of the advances in rheumatoid arthritis therapy. TAA developed in the 1970s with at least 10 designs reported in the literature in that decade.[7] Implant designs included constrained, semiconstrained, and unconstrained designs. Unconstrained designs, relying on ligamentous support, allowed for the greatest freedom of ankle movement, often leading to instability.[8] Early constrained designs imparted forces to the cement-bone interface, resulting in loosening because movement was allowed in only one plane. Current systems permit motion in multiple planes while providing stability.[9,10]

PATIENT SELECTION

No one has yet been able to define precisely the best criteria for determining which patients are best suited for total ankle replacement. Certainly nonoperative care should be tried before any patient becomes a candidate. If the patient does not respond to bracing, physical therapy, or other nonoperative treatment, the patient and surgeon should carefully consider TAA when the ankle joints limits his or her function and causes pain. The ideal patient should be older and have low physical demands, normal body weight, good vascular status, good bone stock, ligamentous integrity, and limited to no hindfoot malalignment.[11] The theory that an older patient is a better candidate than a younger patient is controversial and based on the patient's likely physical demands. The theory assumes that the older patient, who is, let's say, retired and less active than a younger patient, will generate less wear and tear on the device. However, because design options, device materials, and patient activity vary, no one has precisely clarified how to determine the minimum candidate age. Similarly, no one has determined how best to limit candidates by weight. Aside from significant comorbid medical conditions, other problems that typically preclude intervention with TAA include peripheral vascular disease, neuropathy, absent malleoli, severe bone loss, severe deformity, and active infection. Additional absolute contraindications have been significant osteonecrosis of the talus, poor tissue/healing quality, profound malalignment, lower extremity motor dysfunction (eg, Charcot-Marie-Tooth disease, paralysis), and high-demand patients (**Fig. 1**).[12]

Rheumatoid disease is not a contraindication to total ankle replacement. In fact, one study illustrated no statistical difference in implant survival or clinical outcome between rheumatoid and osteoarthritic patients.[13] There is, however, associated perioperative complications, such as wound infections, prosthetic subsidence perhaps due to associated poor bone quality, and aseptic loosening owing to subtalar joint subluxation.[14] An additional concern is the valgus positioning of the ankle, which typically results from rheumatic disease. Deltoid incompetence must be addressed prior to or after ankle replacement to avoid subsequent failure.[15] If the rheumatic disease is longstanding, bony erosions are often identified, furthering valgus, causing deltoid insufficiency, and producing poor bone stock for tibial prosthesis placement.

One should also consider the presence of significant vasculitis and long-term immunosuppressive agents, both of which are linked to wound infection and failure to close.[16] The inflammation associated with rheumatoid arthritis is typically controlled today with corticosteroids and methotrexate. Therefore, perioperative management to avoid adrenal suppression is necessary.[17] Other drugs, such as etanercept, adalimbumab, and infliximab, are "newer" drugs classified at anti–tumor necrosis factor

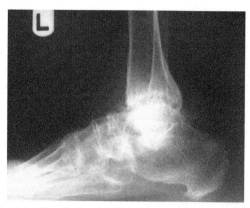

Fig. 1. A preoperative lateral radiograph of a patient with a rheumatoid arthritic ankle.

(TNF). While debate about perioperative management of these drugs goes on, a recent report indicated that continued use of these drugs did not increase the incidence of infection or impaired wound healing.[18]

Other absolute contraindications and relative contraindications depend on the surgeon's experience. Controversy persists about what degree of coronal plane deformity is sufficient as the cutoff for consideration of TAA. Doetz and colleagues[19] found that, during use of mobile-bearing design implants, instability and subluxation of the bearing increases when frontal plane deformity is greater than 10°, leading to failure.[19] They recommended 10° or greater varus or valgus of the ankle or hindfoot as a contraindication to TAA. Hobson and colleagues[20] set 30° of frontal plane deformity to be a contraindication to TAA. Haskell and Mann[21] felt edge loading was 10 times more likely to occur in patients with preoperative incongruent joints as compared with those with congruent joints. The narrowed ankle from the previous fusion requires a smaller implant, which increases stress at the talar component-bone interface, which can lead to loosening, subsidence, and failure.[22] The body mass index relative to the size of the ankle joint is of concern as well. In heavy patients with very small ankle-joint surfaces, increased contact pressures may not be tolerated, leading to poorer outcomes.[23] The use of custom prosthesis components may increase the likelihood of relative contraindications to TAA, such as contraindications involving patients with a high body mass index.[24] Any ipsilateral frontal plane knee deformity should be surgically corrected before TAA because such a deformity will affect the alignment of the ankle and its position relative to the weight-bearing surface. Realignment procedures of the foot at the time of TAA have not been shown to increase incidence of complications.[25]

Patients with rheumatoid arthritis are not immune from complications common to TAA procedures in the general population. Osseous impingement, extra-articular procedures for malalignment, and component replacement occur in the rheumatoid population.[26] Intraoperative and postoperative malleolar fractures, syndesmosis nonunion complications, and wound-healing complications are to be expected, especially early in the learning curve.[27,28] Prosthetic joint infection, when it does occur, is best resolved with a two-stage exchange.[29] Finally, the progressive nature of rheumatoid arthritis and the associated decreased bone mineral density increase the likelihood of periprosthetic osteolysis and implant loosening.

Particle and particulate-induced periprosthetic osteolysis is a major cause of implant loosening and failure.[30] Polyethylene particles in synovial fluid occur in mobile- and fixed-bearing implants in patients undergoing TAA.[31] Wear debris is continually created at the bearing surfaces during motion.[32] Particle concentration and size in TAA are similar to those in total knee arthroplasty as determined by electron microscopy. Particle material, size, shape, and number are factors in tissue reaction to polyethylene and osteolysis. Wear particulates, including polyethylene and metal, induce a chronic inflammatory response at the bone-implant interface. Osteoclasto-genic cytokines RANKL (receptor activator nuclear factor–kappa B ligand), TNF, inter-leukin (IL) 1 (IL-1), IL-6, IL-8, macrophage colony-stimulating factor (M-SCF), and prostaglandin E2 are mediators of particle osteolysis.[30] Theses cytokines also inter-fere with osteogenesis. At the bone-implant interface of a failed total joint arthroplasty, a pseudomembrane forms. This pseudomembrane is composed of fibroblasts, foreign body giant cells, and macrophages. These cells produce IL-6, which induces bone resorption, as well as TNFα and IL-1β. Osteoblasts phagocytose polyethylene and particulate, which significantly increases the secretion of TNFα, IL-6, and RANKL.[33] Fibroblast expression from failed implant biofilm has shown a similar response as synovium from patients without TAA. Angiogenesis is an essential event in the forma-tion and progression of the pseudomembrane.[34] Metal particle exposure to macro-phages results in increased vascular endothelial growth factor, which mediates angiogenesis and osteolysis.[35] This pathologic process is enhanced in the rheumatoid arthritis population, increasing the risk of implant loosening. Radiographic assessment of the talar component can frequently be obscured, making it difficult to assess for periprosthetic lucency. Helical computed tomography with metal-artifact minimization has shown to be more accurate than plain radiographs for early detection and quan-tification of periprosthetic lucency.[36]

The effectiveness of TAA has been reviewed in various studies. Wood and colleagues[37] reviewed 200 TAAs implanted between 2000 and 2003 in a prospective randomized controlled trial of two mobile-bearing implants. The 6-year survival rate was 95 % for the STAR (Scandinavian Total Replacement System) implants (Small Bone Innovations, Inc, Morrisville, PA, USA) and 79% for the Buechel-Pappas implants (Endotec, Inc, South Orange, NJ, USA). Sixty-two of the 200 patients had rheumatoid arthritis. A patient who had a preoperative varus or valgus greater than 15° before surgery was found to have a 6.52 times greater likelihood of developing edge loading. Fourteen (8%) of the 200 TAAs failed and underwent fusion. In two addi-tional studies, Wood and Deakin[38,39] followed the same 200 patients who underwent TAA between 1993 and 2000. One hundred and nineteen patients had inflammatory joint disease, of which 112 were seropositive rheumatoid arthritis. Their 5- and 10-year survival rates were 93.3% and 80.3% respectively. Twenty-four ankles (12%) had been revised, 20 by fusion and 4 by further replacement since the 2000 publica-tion. The investigators did not show TAA to prevent progression of subtalar arthritis. Most patients had preoperative arthritic changes. In their 2000 study, Wood and Deakin commented that it was unlikely that ankle replacement would replace arthrod-esis as has occurred in the knee and that arthrodesis is preferred in patients where heavy and prolonged activity is expected. In their 2008 study, Wood and Deakin antic-ipated that TAA would become as reliable as knee replacement, making it a standard option for the arthritic ankle in the absence of severe frontal plane deformity.

Fevang and colleagues[40] reported on 129 patients with rheumatoid arthritis among 257 patients who underwent TAA.[40] The 5- and 10-year survival rates were 89% and 76% respectively. Two hundred sixteen of the implants were the cementless STAR with three other implants accounting for the remainder of ankles. Twenty-one revisions in the STAR group occurred with 27 (11%) revisions overall. San Giovanni and colleagues[41] reviewed 31 Buechel-Pappas TAAs implanted between 1990 and 1997 in a select low-demand (average age 61 years) patient population with rheumatoid arthritis. The average follow-up was 8.3 years (range 5–12.2 years) with a 93% survival rate and a patient complete satisfaction rate of 83%.[42,43] Two failures resulted in arthrodesis. A prospective study by Doetz and colleagues[19] assessed two cementless mobile-bearing designs in 93 ankles with inflammatory joint disease, mainly rheumatoid arthritis, implanted between 1988 and 1992 (19 ankles) and 1993 to 1999 (74 ankles). The survival rate was 84% at 8 years. Fifteen ankles failed, 13 requiring fusion and 2 resulting in implant exchanges. Seventeen ankles had a preoperative frontal plane deformity of greater than 10°. The 8-year survival rate for this group was 48%. Ankles with less than 10° frontal plane deformity had a survival rate of 90%.

Stengel and colleagues[44] performed a meta-analysis of three-component meniscal-bearing devices that included 1107 TAAs including 415 ankles with rheumatoid arthritis. All but one study used cementless fixation. End-stage rheumatoid arthritis was the leading cause for TAA (37.5%). Superficial infections were 14.5% and 2.5% for retrospective and prospective studies respectively. Deep infections were 3.3% and 0.6% for retrospective and prospective studies respectively. The 5-year survival rate was 90.6%. Revision surgery averaged 12.5% and patients with rheumatoid arthritis had higher incidence of implant loosening and dislocation of components as compared with osteoarthritis and posttraumatic arthritis ankles. The overall range-of-motion improvement was 6.3° (95% CI 2.2–10.5). Su and colleagues[45] reviewed 27 TAAs in patients with rheumatoid arthritis using two different cementless implants (one meniscal-bearing and one two-piece component) between 1988 and 2000. Results were similar between the two systems and, at 6.3 years, 88.5% of the implants were well fixed in stable positions. The postoperative range of motion was greater than 15° arc in all 27 ankles with 17 having greater than 30° of motion. Anderson and colleagues[46] reviewed 51 uncemented STAR TAAs, 28 in patients with rheumatoid arthritis with an average age of 60.5 years. The 5-year survival rate was 70%. Twelve ankles were revised.

Earlier studies are available specific to patients with rheumatoid arthritis. However, they include cemented implants.[3,47] The later generation cemented designs showed a 14-year survival rate of 75.5% in patients with rheumatoid arthritis.[15] Studies

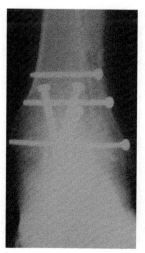

Fig. 2. A rheumatoid patient with an arthritic ankle who underwent a successful ankle arthrodesis.

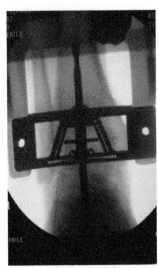

Fig. 3. Intraoperative fluoroscopy is useful to ensure proper alignment of the cutting block.

show a trend of a decreasing survival rates over time for TAAs in the rheumatoid arthritis population. TAA allows for improved walking kinematics as compared with ankle arthrodesis and does not significantly alter mechanical loading of the ankle after ankle replacement.[48] The proprioceptive abilities after TAA do not change when compared with the individual's contralateral side.[49] Studies have not addressed the efficacy of TAA in rheumatoid arthritis patients with severe bone mineral density deficiency.

TOTAL ANKLE ARTHROPLASTY VERSUS ANKLE ARTHRODESIS

Comparison studies provide a unique assessment of TAA and ankle arthrodesis outcomes from within the same surgical groups or centers. Four such studies,

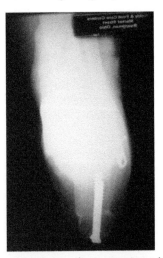

Fig. 4. A postoperative calcaneal axial view demonstrating a lateral calcaneal slide needed for balancing a foot with a calcaneal varus deformity.

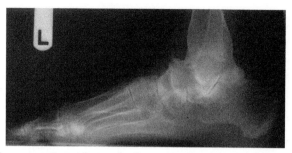

Fig. 5. A lateral preoperative radiograph of a young rheumatoid arthritic patient VO.

including one meta-analysis, are provided. McGuire and colleagues[50] reviewed outcomes comparing the TAA to ankle arthrodesis.[50] TAA was performed in 25 ankles with 10 rheumatoid arthritis ankles in the group. Eighteen patients underwent ankle arthrodesis. Follow-up averaged 3.8 years with an average age of 49.5 years. The arthrodesis group was fused by Charley compression clamp[6,51,52] with interposed iliac bone graft.[7] There was no mention of rheumatoid arthritis patients in this group. Post-traumatic arthrosis,[53–56] failed ankle arthroplasty,[3] and postinfectious arthritis[1] were the indications for ankle arthrodesis. The average age was 41.3 years with an average follow-up of 3.3 years. The arthrodesis group[57,58] had 14 (77%) excellent, 3 (16%) good, 0 fair, 0 poor, and 1 (6%) failed results. The arthroplasty group[13] had 9 (36%) excellent, 9 (36%) good, 0 fair, 2 poor, and 5 (20%) failed results. Koefoed and Stürup[59] performed a prospective study comparing 14 ankle arthrodeses to 14 TAAs.[59] The average age was 54 years (range 27–71 years) and 39 years (range 21–68 years) for the TAA and ankle arthrodesis groups respectively. The average age for the arthritis subset groups was 48 years (range 45–50 years) and 24 years (range 21–31 years) for the TAA and ankle arthrodesis groups respectively. Four ankles in each group had rheumatoid arthritis. All surgeries were performed between 1981 and 1985. Median follow-up was 84 months. Arthrodeses were performed with

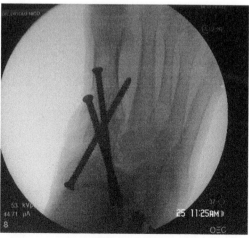

Fig. 6. An intraoperative anterior-posterior view of a medial column stabilization before implantation of a prosthesis (a staged surgery) in patient VO.

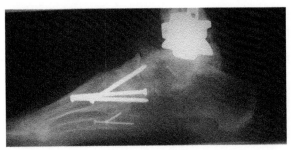

Fig. 7. A 7-year postoperative lateral radiograph of patient VO post–medial column stabilization (a staged surgery) followed by insertion of an Agility ankle prostheses (DePuy Orthopaedics, Inc, Warsaw, IN, USA).

a Charnley frame and arthroplasty was performed with a two-piece cemented implant. The ankle arthrodesis group had four deep infections, three nonunions, and five cases where subtalar arthrosis developed. The TAA group had no deep infections, three cases of skin necrosis, one revisional arthrodesis, and no development of subtalar arthrosis. Investigators found that those in the arthroplasty group experienced better pain relief, higher levels of function, and lower infection rates without the development of subtalar arthritis (**Fig. 2**).

Soohoo and colleagues[60] compared reoperation rates between 4705 ankle arthrodeses and 480 ankle replacements during a 10-year study period from 1995 to 2004. Six percent of the ankle fusion patients and 10 percent of the TAA patients had rheumatoid arthritis. Rates of revision surgery were 9% at 1 year and 23% at 5 years in the TAA group. Corresponding rates of revision in the arthrodesis group were 5% and 11%. Patients who had an ankle arthrodesis had a 2.8% occurrence of subtalar fusion at 5 years as compared with a TAA rate of 0.7%. Regression analysis confirmed a significant increase in the risk of major revision surgery in the TAA group.

Saltzman and colleagues[61] performed a nonrandomized study with concurrent controls as part of a Food and Drug Administration (FDA) study to evaluate the safety and efficacy of the STAR implant to treat arthritis. The pivotal STAR group included

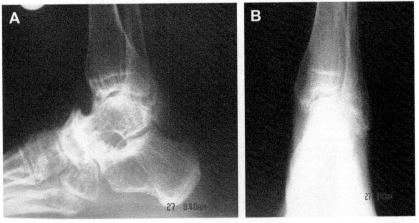

Fig. 8. Anterior-posterior (*A*) and lateral (*B*) radiographs of a rheumatoid arthritic ankle and talar-navicular joint of patient TZ.

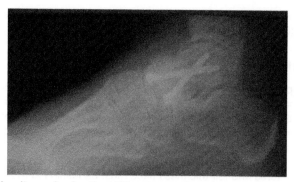

Fig. 9. A lateral radiograph of patient TZ postoperative talar-navicular arthrodesis (staged surgery) before implantation of prosthesis.

158 ankles and the pivotal fusion group included 66 ankles. A continued access STAR group (N = 435) was evaluated also. Patients with rheumatoid arthritis accounted for 12.7% of the STAR group and 6.5 % of the fusion group. The pivotal groups were similar in gender, race, height, and weight. With the exception of pain and an expected loss of motion in the fusion group, operative site adverse events were higher in the STAR pivotal group. These events included nerve injury, bone fracture, edema, wound problems, and bony changes. Major complications, with the exception of infection, were also higher in the STAR group. The STAR group performed better in most functional scoring subscales except for pain relief, walking, and the presence of a limp.

Haddad and colleagues,[62,63] in a systematic review of the literature, compared 852 TAAs to 1262 ankle arthrodeses. Fifty-six percent of the arthrodesis studies were published between 1990 and 1997 and all of the TAA studies were published between 1998 and 2005. Follow-up was 2 to 9 years for the TAA group and 2 to 23 years in the arthrodesis group. Results in the TAA group were 38% excellent, 30.5% good, 5.5% fair, and 24% poor with a 7% revision rate. Five- and 10-year survival rates were 78% and 77% respectively. The corresponding results in the arthrodesis group

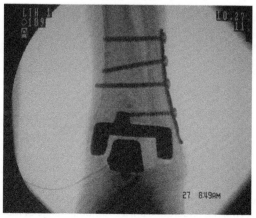

Fig. 10. Intraoperative anterior-posterior view of patient TZ following implantation of an Agility prostheses.

were 31%, 37%, 13%, and 13% with a 9% revision rate. The main reason for revision was nonunion (65%).

SURGICAL TECHNIQUE

There is a steep learning curve with TAA as it is probably one of the most technically demanding procedures performed in the foot and ankle.[25] Most of the current FDA-approved prostheses use an anterior approach. This approach requires an extensive incision and it must be handled with great respect. The incision is made between the tibialis anterior and the extensor hallucis longus tendons. The anterior neurovascular structures should be recognized and retracted laterally. The incision is carried down to the bony structures and full-thickness flaps must be fashioned to avoid undermining. The incision needs to be sufficiently long to prevent needless tension while retracting.

Balancing of the foot and ankle should be performed with ligament tension or loosening (if not already addressed with a prior surgery) through a variety of techniques. To address ankle instability, this balancing may include a lateral ankle stabilization procedure, which may require, for example, a midfoot arthodesis in the case of a collapsed midfoot. Failure to address ankle instability will likely lead to a failed TAA. Subsequent

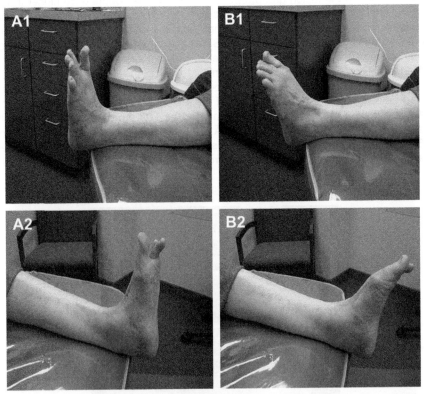

Fig. 11. Clinical postoperative view of extension (*A1* and *A2*) and flexion (*B1* and *B2*) of a rheumatoid patient who has undergone a TAA. Although range of motion postoperatively is limited, the range of motion is greater than what it was preoperatively and the motion is pain-free.

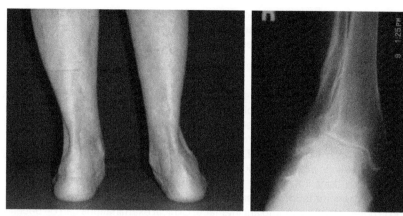

Fig. 12. A clinical and radiographic view of a prospective TAA patient. Consideration is needed for balancing the foot and ankle before implantation. Lengthening on the fibula and a supramalleolar osteotomy would be indicated before implantation.

to balancing of the foot and ankle, the ankle is prepared for bone cuts. All of the current FDA prostheses use an alignment guide and cutting block. It is essential to use intra-operative fluoroscopy to line up the cutting jig for suitable placement of the prostheses. It is crucial for the surgeon to be conscious of the posterior medial tendons and neurovascular structures of the posterior medial ankle as these structures are easily visible once the tibial bone cut is resected. Once the bone cuts are complete, a trial prosthesis is inserted and viewed both clinically and radiographically. The proper size is determined and inserted. Frequently following a TAA, a gastrocnemius recession or an Achilles tendon lengthening may be needed for a tight posterior

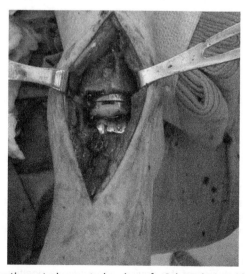

Fig. 13. An intraoperative anterior-posterior view of a Salto Talaris ankle prosthesis (Tornier, Minneapolis, MN, USA). Note the long expansile full-thickness incision to decrease tension on the soft tissue envelope.

muscle group. Careful soft tissue closure is performed to avoid unnecessary tension. A closed suction drain is typically used and it is imperative that the soft tissues are handled delicately to avoid postoperative soft tissue complications (**Figs. 3–13**).

POSTOPERATIVE COURSE

Typically a drain is used and removed approximately 3 days postoperatively. Sutures can be removed at 2 to 3 weeks. Following the below-the-knee casting, the patient is placed in a walking boot and prescribed physical therapy for 1 to 2 months. The protocol of the authors is 6 weeks of strict non–weight bearing in a below-the-knee cast for all implants except the STAR. The STAR implant patients are non–weight bearing for 2 weeks in a below-the-knee cast. The prosthesis relies on bony in-growth at the prosthesis-bone interface.

The authors recommend serial ankle radiographs every 2 to 3 weeks until good bonding is noted at the bone-implant interface. Clinical examinations can be deceiving and may not correlate with radiographic changes. Weight-bearing and non–weight-bearing views should be routinely taken.[64] The latter should be taken while maximally dorsiflexing and plantarflexing for evaluation of range of motion. Any angular change greater than 5° in either component suggests subsidence or implant migration.[9] Loosening of the talar component should be considered if comparative lateral views illustrate more than 5-mm subsidence.[46] Radiolucency around an implant can be also a sign of loosening and 2 mm is considered significant.[65] Correlate these findings to operative and postoperative views to ensure radiolucency is not a result of surgical technique. In cases of concern, computerized tomography has been shown to be superior to radiographs for periprosthetic radiolucencies.[36]

COMPLICATIONS

Wound healing with ankle replacement procedures are well documented in the literature. The surrounding tissues can be frail and closer to bone, making resistance to edema and tissue strain difficult, especially in rheumatoid patients. Complications related to wound healing have been reported in up to 40% of cases.[66] Wound dehiscence can be counteracted by minimizing edema, through leg elevation and the use of firm compression bandages, and by offsetting hematoma formation, through the use of drains (**Figs. 14** and **15**).[67]

Thromboembolism is a highly debated topic amongst foot and ankle surgeons. The authors have found no literature that suggests rheumatoid disease increases risk of deep vein thrombosis. However, surgeries over 30 minutes, hypertension, history of deep vein thrombosis, smoking, prolonged postoperative immobilization, stroke, oral contraceptives, obesity, age older than 40 years, diabetes, and other factors have been linked to increased risk of thromboembolism.[68] The medical literature does not support mandatory routine prophylaxis in patients undergoing foot and ankle surgery.[69] However, mechanical methods, such as sequential compression device or compression stockings, are recommended.[69]

Malleolar fractures are the most frequent complication during surgery, the most at risk being the medial malleolus.[19] To reduce the risk for this complication, some suggest that the medial malleolus be pinned before any osteotomy is made. This should prevent excursion of the saw blade and overzealous cuts.[17]

Malalignment can of course occur in not just one plane, but in multiple planes. Placement of the jig, design of the device, varus/valgus positioning, lateral/medial/anterior/posterior positioning, and improper sizing of the implant have all been implicated in malalignment.[28] Distraction can be a potential danger. Too little distraction

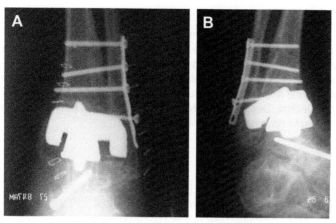

Fig. 14. A complication involving a medial malleolus fracture and tibial component subsidence.

can result in "stuffing" the joint with the prosthesis, leading to pain and limited range of motion.

Infection, particularly in patients who have rheumatoid arthritis with immunosuppression, is a major concern. These infections can be classified into two types: superficial and deep. Early and prompt treatment is necessary to stop the infection before it reaches a stage requiring removal of components. Aseptic loosening and osteolysis are possible in total ankle replacements. It is extremely important for the surgeon to ensure that components have good cortical support. Without good cortical support, soft cancellous bone inevitably subsides. The level of the tibial resection is determined to generate sufficient room for the components and restore length and tension to the ligaments.

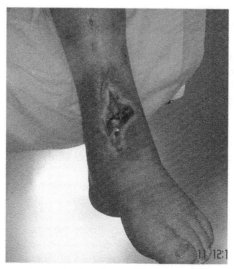

Fig. 15. Clinical view of a rheumatoid patient with implant exposure and a large wound dehiscence.

SUMMARY

Total ankle replacement in the rheumatoid patient is feasible and effective treatment for ankle arthritis. The benefits of ankle prosthesis are good pain relief, acceptable function, and patient satisfaction. It is a joint-sparing procedure to restore functionality. All investigators of total ankle replacement feel that, as clinicians gain experience with the procedure and related products, difficulties and risks associated with the procedure will decline. Despite an early history of failure and poor patient satisfaction, more recent results have shown promise.

REFERENCES

1. Lorenzo M. Rheumatoid arthritis. Foot Ankle Clin 2007;12:525–37.
2. Spiegel TM, Spiegel JS. Rheumatoid arthritis in the foot and ankle: diagnosis, pathology, and treatment. Foot Ankle 1982;2:318–24.
3. Lachiewicz P, Inglis A, Ranawat C. Total ankle replacement in rheumatoid arthritis. J Bone Joint Surg Am 1984;66(3):340–3.
4. Michelson J, Easley M, Wigley FM. Foot and ankle problems in rheumatoid arthritis. Foot Ankle 1994;15:608–13.
5. Jaakkola JI, Mann RA. A review of rheumatoid arthritis affecting the foot and ankle. Foot Ankle Int 2004;25(12):866–74.
6. Pyevich M, Saltzman C, Callaghan J, et al. Total ankle arthroplasty: a unique design. Two to twelve year follow-up. J Bone Joint Surg Am 1998;80(10):1410–20.
7. Gougoulias N, Khanna A, Maffulli N. History and evolution in total ankle arthroplasty. Br Med Bull 2009;89:111–51.
8. Castro M. Ankle Biomechanics. Foot Ankle Clin N Am 2002;7:679–93.
9. Valderrabano V, Hinterman B, Dick W. Scandinavian total ankle replacement. A 3.7-year average followup of 65 patients. Clin Orthop Relat Res 2004;424:47–56.
10. Lord G, Marrotte JH. Total ankle prosthesis. Technique and first results. Apropos of 12 cases. Rev Chir Orthop Reparatrice Appar Mot 1973;59:139–51.
11. Clare MP, Sanders RW. Preoperative considerations in ankle replacement surgery. Foot Ankle Clin 2002;7:709–20.
12. Hintermann B, Valderrabano V. Total ankle replacement. Foot Ankle Clin 2003;8: 375–405.
13. Kofoed H, Sorensen TS. Ankle arthroplasty for rheumatoid arthritis and osteoarthritis: prospective long term study of cemented replacements. J Bone Joint Surg Br 1998;80:328–32.
14. Alvine FG. Total ankle arthroplasty. In: Myerson MS, editor. Foot and ankle disorders. 1st edition. Philadelphia: WB Saunders; 2000. p. 1085–102.
15. Neufeld SK, Lee TH. Total ankle arthroplasty: indications, results, and biomechanical rationale. Am J Orthop 2000;29:593–602.
16. Newton SE III. Total ankle arthroplasty: clinical study of fifty cases. J Bone Joint Surg Am 1982;62:104–11.
17. Wood PL, Crawford LA, Suneja R, et al. Total ankle replacement for rheumatoid ankle arthritis. Foot Ankle Clin 2007;12:497–508.
18. Bibbo C, Goldberg JW. Infections and healing complications after elective orthopedic foot and ankle surgery during tumor necrosis factor–alpha inhibition therapy. Foot Ankle Int 2004;25(5):331–5.
19. Doets HC, Brand R, Nelissen RG. Total ankle arthroplasty in inflammatory joint disease with use of two mobile bearing designs. J Bone Joint Surg Am 2006; 88(6):1272–84.

20. Hobson A, Karantana A, Dhar S. Total ankle replacement in patients with significant pre-operative deformity of the hindfoot. J Bone Joint Surg Br 2009;91(4): 481–6.
21. Haskell A, Mann R. Ankle arthroplasty with preoperative coronal plane deformity. Short term results. Clin Orthop Relat Res 2004;424:98–103.
22. Hintermann B, Barg A, Knupp M, et al. Conversion of painful ankle arthrodesis to total ankle arthroplasty. J Bone Joint Surg Am 2009;91:850–8.
23. Nicholson J, Parks B, Stroud C, et al. Joint characteristics in agility total ankle arthroplasty. Clin Orthop Relat Res 2004;424:125–9.
24. Myerson M, Won H. Primary and revision total ankle replacement using custom-designed prostheses. Foot Ankle Clin N Am 2008;13:521–38.
25. Schuberth J, Patel S, Zarutsky E. Perioperative complications of the agility total ankle replacement in 50 initial, consecutive cases. J Foot Ankle Surg 2006; 45(3):139–46.
26. Spirt A, Assal M, Hansen S. Complications and failure after total ankle arthroplasty. J Bone Joint Surg Am 2004;86(6):1172–8.
27. McGarvey W, Clanton T, Lunz D. Malleolar fracture after total ankle arthroplasty. Clin Orthop Relat Res 2004;424:104–10.
28. Conti SF, Wong YS. Complications of total ankle replacement. Foot Ankle Clin 2002;7:791–807.
29. Berbari E, Osmon D, Duffy M, et al. Outcome of prosthetic joint infection in patients with rheumatoid arthritis: the impact of medical and surgical therapy in 200 episodes. Clin Infect Dis 2006;42(2):216–23.
30. Yamanaka Y, Abu-Amer W, Foglia D, et al. NFAT2 is an essential mediator of orthopedic particle-induced osteoclastogenesis. J Orthop Res 2008;26:1577–84.
31. Kobayashi A, Minoda Y, Kadoya Y, et al. Ankle arthroplasties generate wear particles similar to knee arthroplasties. Clin Orthop Relat Res 2004;424:69–72.
32. Tuan R, Lee F, Konttinen Y, et al. What are the local and systemic biologic reactions and mediators to wear debris, and what host factors determine or modulate the biologic response to wear? J Am Acad Orthop Surg 2008;16(Suppl 1):S42–8.
33. Koreny T, Tunyogi-Csapo M, Gal I, et al. The role of fibroblast-derived factors in periprosthetic osteolysis. Arthritis Rheum 2006;54(10):3221–32.
34. Tunyogi-Csapo M, Koreny T, Vermes C, et al. The role of fibroblasts-derived growth factors in periprosthetic angiogenesis. J Orthop Relat Res 2007;25:1378–88.
35. Miyanishi K, Trindade C, Ma T, et al. Periprosthetic osteolysis: induction of vascular endothelial growth factor from human monocyte/macrophages by orthopaedic biomaterial particles. J Bone Miner Res 2003;18(9):1573–83.
36. Hanna R, Haddad S, Lazarus M. Evaluation of periprosthetic lucency after total ankle arthroplasty: helical CT versus conventional radiography. Foot Ankle Int 2007;28(8):921–6.
37. Wood P, Sutton C, Mishra V, et al. A randomized, controlled trial of two mobile-bearing total ankle replacements. J Bone Joint Surg Br 2009;91:69–74.
38. Wood P, Deakin S. Total ankle replacement. The results in 200 ankles. J Bone Joint Surg Br 2003;85:334–41.
39. Wood P, Prem H, Sutton C. Total ankle replacement. Medium-term results in 200 Scandinavian total ankle replacements. J Bone Joint Surg Br 2008;90:605–9.
40. Fevang B, Lie S, Havelin L. 257 Ankle arthroplasties performed in Norway between 1994 and 2005. Acta Orthop 2007;78(5):575–83.
41. San Giovanni T, Keblish D, Thomas W, et al. Eight-year results of a minimally constrained total ankle arthroplasty. Foot Ankle Int 2006;27(6):418–26.

42. Eppeland S, Mykelbust G, Hodt-Billington C, et al. Gait patterns in subjects with rheumatoid arthritis cannot be explained by reduced speed alone. Gait Posture 2009;29:499–503.

43. Piriou P, Culpan P, Mullins M, et al. Ankle replacement versus arthrodesis: a comparative gait analysis study. Foot Ankle Int 2008;29(1):3–9.

44. Stengel D, Bauwens K, Ekkernkamp A. Efficacy of total ankle replacement with meniscal-bearing devices: a systematic review and meta-analysis. Arch Orthop Trauma Surg 2005;125:109–19.

45. Su E, Kahn B, Figgie M. Total ankle replacement in patients with rheumatoid arthritis. Clin Orthop Relat Res 2004;424:32–8.

46. Anderson T, Montgomery F, Carlsson A. Uncemented STAR total ankle prosthesis: three to eight year follow up of fifty one consecutive ankles. J Bone Joint Surg Am 2003;85:1321–9.

47. Unger A, Inglis A, Mow C, et al. Total ankle arthroplasty in rheumatoid arthritis: a long term follow-up study. Foot Ankle 1998;8(4):173–9.

48. Houdjik H, Doets H, van Middlekoop M, et al. Joint stiffness of the ankle during walking after successful mobile-bearing total ankle replacement. Gait Posture 2008;27:115–9.

49. Conti S, Dazen D, Stewart G, et al. Proprioception after total ankle arthroplasty. Foot Ankle Int 2008;29(11):1069–73.

50. McGuire M, Kyle R, Gustilo R, et al. Comparative analysis of ankle arthroplasty versus ankle arthrodesis. Clin Orthop Relat Res 1988;226:174–81.

51. Pappas M, Buechel FF, DePalma AF. Cylindrical total ankle joint replacement: surgical and biomechanical rationale. Clin Orthop 1976;118:82–92.

52. Rippstein PF. Clinical experiences with three different designs of ankle prostheses. Foot Ankle Clin 2002;7:817–31.

53. Nishikawa M, Tomita T, Fujii M, et al. Total ankle replacement in rheumatoid arthritis. Int Orthop 2004;28:123–6.

54. Hvid I, Rasmussen O, Jensen N, et al. Trabecular bone strength profiles at the ankle joint. Clin Orthop Relat Res 1985;199:306–12.

55. Henne TD, Anderson JG. Total ankle arthroplasty: a historical perspective. Foot Ankle Clin 2002;7:695–702.

56. Evanski PH, Waugh TR. Management of arthritis of the ankle, an alternative to arthrodesis. Clin Orthop 1977;122:110–5.

57. Haider H. Fixed or mobile bearing total ankle replacement designs: What really matters? Invited Talk. Toronto (ON): Inbone Technologies Educational Event; 2007.

58. Guyer AJ, Richardson EG. Current concepts review: total ankle arthroplasty. Foot Ankle Int 2008;29(2):256–64.

59. Koefoed H, Stürup J. Comparison of ankle arthroplasty and arthrodesis. A prospective series with long term follow-up. Foot 1994;4:6–9.

60. SooHoo N, Zingmond D, Ko C. Comparison of reoperation rates following ankle arthrodesis and total ankle arthroplasty. J Bone Joint Surg Am 2007;89:2143–9.

61. Saltzman C, Mann R, Ahrens J, et al. Prospective controlled trial of STAR total ankle replacement versus ankle fusion: initial results. Foot Ankle Int 2009;30(7): 579–93.

62. Haddad S, Coetzee J, Estok R, et al. Intermediate and long-term outcomes of total ankle arthroplasty and ankle arthrodesis. J Bone Joint Surg Am 2007;89: 1899–905.

63. Bestic JM, Peterson JJ, DeOrio JK, et al. Postoperative evaluation of the total ankle arthroplasty. AJR Am J Roentgenol 2008;190:1112–22.

64. Berquist TH, DeOrio JK. Reconstructive procedures. In: Berquist TH, editor. Radiology of the foot and ankle. 2nd edition. Philadelphia: Lippencott Williams & Wilkins; 2000. p. 479–85.
65. Bolton-Maggs BG, Sudlow SA, Freeman MA, et al. Total ankle arthroplasty, a long term review of the London hospital experience. J Bone Joint Surg 1985;67(5): 785–90.
66. Bibbo C. Wound healing complications and infection following surgery for rheumatoid arthritis. Foot Ankle Clin 2007;12:509–24.
67. Slaybaugh RS, Beasley BD, Massa EG. Deep venous thrombosis risk assessment, incidence, and prophylaxis in foot and ankle surgery. Clin Podiatr Med Surg 2003;20:269–89.
68. Wukich DK, Waters DH. Thromboembolism following foot and ankle surgery: a case series and literature review. J Foot Ankle Surg 2008;47(3):243–9.
69. Geerts WH, Pinco GF, Heit JA, et al. Prevention of venous thromboembolism: the seventh ACCP conference on antithrombic and thrombolytic therapy. Chest 2004; 126(Suppl 3):338s–400s.

The Complications Encountered with the Rheumatoid Surgical Foot and Ankle

Christopher L. Reeves, DPM, FACFAS[a,b,*], Adam J. Peaden, DPM[a,c],
Amber M. Shane, DPM, FACFAS[a,d]

KEYWORDS

• Rheumatoid • Arthritis • Complications • Surgical

Complications are an inevitable obstacle in many surgical procedures involving the foot and ankle and seem to be especially unavoidable in patients with rheumatoid arthritis (RA). Approximately 0.5% to 1% of the population has RA, and up to 90% of those afflicted with RA will have manifestations of the disease in the foot and ankle.[1,2] When nonsurgical measures for treating the disease's manifestations in the foot and ankle are exhausted, surgical options must be considered but only with a firm understanding of the disease process and the complications that may arise.

RA is a chronic, degenerative, systemic disease that leads to the destruction of articular cartilage of the joints via deposition of immunoglobulins, rheumatoid factors, and immune complexes into the joint synovium, causing an inflammatory response in the joint tissues. This in turn leads to synovial hyperplasia and angiogenesis. Interleukin-1 and tumor necrosis factor stimulate the inflamed synovium to produce proteolytic enzymes (collagenase and streptolysin) that attack the joints, eroding the articular cartilage and the surrounding bone. Local osteopenia is caused by the increased blood flow to the synovial tissues.[3] This autoimmune response and

[a] Department of Podiatric Surgery (East Orlando Campus), Florida Hospital East Orlando, 7975 Lake Underhill Road, Suite 210, Orlando, FL 32822, USA
[b] Orlando Foot and Ankle Clinic, 25 West Kaley Street, Suite 300, Orlando, FL 32806, USA
[c] Department of Medical Education, Florida Hospital East Orlando, 7975 Lake Underhill Road, Suite 210, Orlando, FL 32822, USA
[d] Orlando Foot and Ankle Clinic, 250 North Alafaya Trail, Orlando, FL 32828, USA
* Corresponding author. Orlando Foot and Ankle Clinic, 25 West Kaley Street, Suite 300, Orlando, FL 32806.
E-mail address: Docreeves1@yahoo.com

Clin Podiatr Med Surg 27 (2010) 313–325
doi:10.1016/j.cpm.2009.12.002
0891-8422/10/$ – see front matter © 2010 Published by Elsevier Inc.

podiatric.theclinics.com

impending osseous weakening promote an environment that can easily lead to both soft tissue and osseous complications.

Many complications, including infection, delays in wound healing, malunion, nonunion, implant failure, and degeneration of adjacent joints soon after primary fusion, have been described in the literature and are generally accepted as commonplace in reconstructive surgeries of the foot and ankle.[4] Rheumatoid patients typically have osteopenia, making rigid internal fixation a challenge. Minor vasculitis combined with weak, friable skin complicates wound healing.[3] Because of the nature of the disease, many patients undergo multiple surgeries for the correction of subsequent deformities. This makes anatomic dissection a challenge, thereby increasing the trauma to the surrounding tissues, once again increasing the risk of surgical-site complications. There is also a common belief that disease-modifying pharmaceuticals and immunosuppressive therapy modalities that are commonly used in patients with RA increase the risk of infection. However, this has been refuted in many recent studies addressing this specific topic.[5,6]

WOUND HEALING AND INFECTION

Wound healing problems by far are the most commonly described complications in rheumatoid foot and ankle surgery throughout the literature. Some investigators have described delayed healing as a "relative complication" that should be expected and considered a part of the normal postoperative course.[4] A 2003 study by Bibbo and colleagues[7] reported on 104 rheumatoid patients who were undergoing 725 procedures; the overall complication rate was 32%, with wound healing problems as the most common complication followed by superficial infections, nonunion, and delayed union. Other studies have listed wound healing problems in the range of 4% to 24% and infection rates in the range of 0% to 14%.[8–13]

If a deep infection occurs postoperatively and there is a suspicion of bone infection, hardware should be removed as soon as possible and a bone biopsy should be performed to definitively determine the presence of osteomyelitis. If bone infection is indeed present, the use of external fixation may prove beneficial to maintain bony alignment while antibiotic spacers and intravenous antibiotics are used to treat the infection. Further internal fixation could be used after infection is no longer present with bone biopsy.

PREOPERATIVE EVALUATION

When comparing the overall infection and delayed wound healing rates of approximately 1.5% in all elective foot and ankle surgeries[14] with the statistics listed earlier for patients with RA, the approach to the rheumatoid foot and ankle surgical patient must be a cautious one. As with all patients, but especially in a patient with poor skin quality and questionable vascular status, a thorough vascular evaluation must be performed. Without a sufficient vascular supply, wound healing will undoubtedly be delayed, if not impossible. Nonpalpable pedal pulses, decreased hair growth on the lower legs, and diminished capillary refill time are all indications for further noninvasive arterial analysis. Ankle-brachial indices and segmental pressures may point to arterial disease and provide a good screening tool for vascular insufficiency. Further invasive vascular workup, such as an arteriogram with subsequent arterial stenting or bypass surgery, may be necessary and is best performed by a vascular surgeon. A patient with suspected vascular insufficiency undergoing digital surgery would benefit from analysis of the toe pressures. Toe pressures should be greater than 40 mm Hg with pulsatile waveforms. Venous evaluation is much more rudimentary but is also important. A patient with poor venous outflow will be at greater risk for increased edema postoperatively, which could also lead to wound dehiscence and increased pain. These studies should not be the only evaluation tool and should not replace overall clinical suspicion of vascular insufficiency in the rheumatoid patient. If there is any question, appropriate vascular consults should be obtained.

PERIOPERATIVE MEDICATION MANAGEMENT

In the past, rheumatologists have recommended temporary discontinuation of the use of antirheumatic medications, including nonsteroidal antiinflammatory drugs (NSAIDs), corticosteroids, methotrexate, gold, and anti–TNF-α agents, to minimize the risk of postoperative healing complications. This has been shown in a multitude of studies to be unnecessary.[3] Several disadvantages to this approach have been discussed in the literature. It is suspected that discontinuation of anti-TNF treatments may elicit an increase in disease activity and that increases in corticosteroid doses in the perioperative course may increase the risk of infection. Also, long-term interruptions in anti-TNF medications may cause an antibody response, leading to infusion reactions and ineffectiveness of presurgical doses in the future.[15] A host of studies have shown that discontinuation of these RA medications in the perioperative period have made no significant difference in operative outcomes. A 2001 study[16] of 388 patients with RA who underwent elective orthopedic procedures divided patients into 3 groups: Group A consisted of those who continued methotrexate throughout the perioperative period; Group B consisted of those who discontinued methotrexate 2 weeks before surgery; and Group C consisted of 288 patients who were never prescribed methotrexate. Infections or surgical complications were observed in 2 patients of 88 in Group A (2%), 11 of 72 in Group B (15%), and 24 of 288 in Group C (10.5%). A 2003 study by Bibbo and colleagues[17] analyzed the results of 725 foot and ankle procedures in 104 patients with RA with an overall complication rate of 32%. The authors found that the use of methotrexate, steroids, gold, NSAIDs, or hydroxychloroquine had no contribution to the development of postoperative healing or infectious complications. Furthermore, they found that the presence of rheumatoid nodules was not a predictor of postoperative complications as previously suspected. Bibbo and Goldberg's[18] study on TNF-α inhibitors in 2004 found that the patients who continued the medication throughout the perioperative period had fewer total complications than those who did not receive the drugs in the same period. A similar study of 768 patients with RA who underwent 1219 orthopedic procedures demonstrated complication rates of 8.7% in those who received anti–TNF-α medications, 4% in those who did not receive the medications, and 5.8% in those who discontinued the medications in the perioperative period.[15] This further supports the continued use of rheumatoid medications throughout the perioperative course.

Antibiotics should be used in all rheumatoid patients undergoing foot and ankle surgery. First generation cephalosporins, such as cefazolin (or clindamycin in the penicillin allergic patient), should always be used.[19] Infectious disease specialists may recommend methicillin-resistant *Staphylococcus aureus* (MRSA) coverage with intravenous vancomycin in the patient who has had previous colonization, and some even recommend nasal mupirocin and chlorhexidine baths 5 days preoperatively in patients with MRSA-positive nasal cultures.[20]

INTRAOPERATIVE CONSIDERATIONS

Rheumatoid foot and ankle deformities are often severe and long-standing, thus leading to significant soft tissue adaptation and contractures. As a result, acute correction of a chronic deformity in the rheumatoid foot may lead to many complications, including digital ischemia caused by small vessel kinking and stretching and the inability to close surgical wounds in the traditional manner. For instance, correction of a severe calcaneal valgus deformity with a lateral incision for triple arthrodesis may require careful incision planning because the heel will be brought out of its valgus position into a more rectus position, causing gapping or tension at the incision site when closed primarily. A pie-crusting technique may be used in this situation to reduce the excess skin tension (**Fig. 1**). Careful surgical incision placement is vital. For example, during a pan metatarsal head resection in which a plantar incision is utilized it is important ensure that the wedge of skin excised is oriented to avoid excessive pressure and protect against wound gapping (**Fig. 2**). The surgeon must have additional closure techniques in their armamentarium such as the ability to perform rotation flaps or have plastic surgical services available when performing reconstructive foot and ankle surgery. Vacuum-assisted closure therapy may be used in those instances in which primary closure is unobtainable. Protection of the soft tissue envelope through careful anatomic dissection and delicate tissue handling must always be performed. A compressive dressing placed on the extremity to decrease edema postoperatively can decrease the risk of wound dehiscence.

POSTOPERATIVE CARE

Intravenous antibiotics should be continued for at least 3 additional doses if the patient is to remain in the hospital for observation.[14] In conjunction with compressive dressings, edema can best be controlled by limiting the patients' activity and by limb elevation. Oxygen via a nasal cannula may be used postoperatively in patients at high risk for vascular compromise, and restriction of nicotine and caffeine is recommended to reduce the risk of arterial constriction. Segmental compression devices and low-molecular-weight heparin should be used for approximately 14 days after surgery for the prevention of deep vein thrombosis.[14] The first postoperative office visit may be scheduled sooner than for the average patient because the risk of wound dehiscence and infection may be higher.

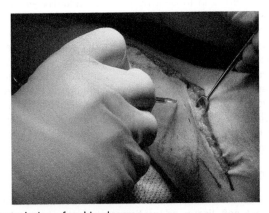

Fig. 1. Pie-crusting technique for skin closure.

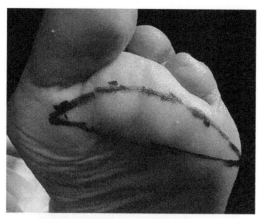

Fig. 2. Plantar incision for panmetatarsal head resection.

COMPLICATIONS IN FOREFOOT SURGERY

Deformities in the forefoot are a common source of pain in patients with RA. Chronic inflammation in the metatarsophalangeal (MP) joints leads to capsular laxity and imbalances between the extrinsic and intrinsic musculatures of the foot.[21] Hammering of the digits occurs that may cause painful plantar callosities or ulceration in the patient with neuropathic RA (**Figs. 3** and **4**). The incidence of hallux abducto valgus in the rheumatoid foot ranges between 59% and 90% in the literature, most likely as a result of chronic inflammation leading to capsular imbalances and destruction of the bony structure of the first metatarsal head.[3] First MP joint arthrodesis, first MP joint implant arthroplasty, panmetatarsal head resection, and digital fusion are the common surgical approaches to provide pain relief in severe deformities.

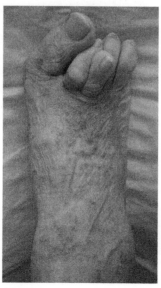

Fig. 3. Rheumatoid forefoot deformity.

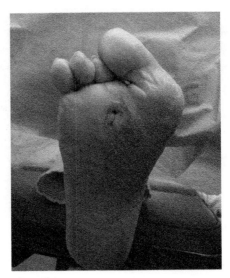

Fig. 4. Plantar forefoot ulceration.

Digital deformity is a common occurrence in the rheumatoid foot, and proximal interphalangeal joint fusion is commonly performed along with adjunct procedures, such as MP joint capsulotomy and extensor tenotomy. These procedures can effectively decrease the pressure at the distal aspect of the toe and also relieve pain caused

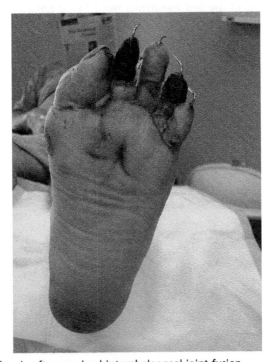

Fig. 5. Digital ischemia after proximal interphalangeal joint fusion.

by dorsal calluses at the proximal interphalangeal joints. However, digits are at very high risk for vascular embarrassment because of the nature of the surgery, with stretching and kinking of the vessels commonly occurring in the correction of severe deformity (**Fig. 5**).

Panmetatarsal head resection is one of the most rudimentary procedures for the painful forefoot with metatarsalgia and digital deformities, with the intent of the surgery based on pain relief. McGarvey and Johnson[22] studied 49 panmetatarsal head resections with wire stabilization across the first metatarsophalangeal (MP) joint. With an average follow-up of almost 5 years, first MP joint pain and recurrent deformity with persistent metatarsalgia were noted in 53% of patients. Cavanagh and colleagues[23] studied forefoot pressures in 2 diabetic patients before and after panmetatarsal head resection and noted that despite the removal of all of the metatarsal heads, new focal regions of increased pressure appeared in gait studies and ulceration occurred in one of the patients after the occurrence of ectopic bone growth at the level of the metatarsal head resection.

First MP joint arthrodesis is also a common approach and is discussed frequently in the literature. Coughlin[24] reported on a series of patients undergoing first MP joint arthrodesis, with lesser metatarsal head resection in 32 patients (47 feet) who had dorsal plating systems with a single compression screw. A 100% fusion rate was reported, and redislocation was noted in only 13 of the 132 toes that were dislocated preoperatively (10%). Ectopic bone formation was noted in 8% of the lesser metatarsals. One ischemic toe was noted. Smith and colleagues[25] reported on 26 first MP joint arthrodeses using threaded K wires, with a fusion rate of 96% and with 1 asymptomatic pseudoarthrosis, no infections, and no reoperations. Mann and Thompson[26] performed the same operation on 18 feet with only 1 nonunion. The authors later reported in a study on the same patients that hallux interphalangeal joint arthritis was noted on plain radiographs in 65% of the patients, but all were asymptomatic.[27]

Preservation of the first MP joint has also been reported in the literature. Thordarson and colleagues[21] reported on 8 patients (15 feet) with forefoot deformities and RA, 13 of which underwent joint preservation surgery for hallux valgus via chevron osteotomies in 8 feet, chevron and Akin osteotomies in 1 foot, and hallux interphalangeal joint fusion in 2 feet because the metatarsal head did not seem eroded. Two of the 15 patients underwent fusion of the first MP joint. The 2 remaining patients underwent fewer toe procedures because their first MP joints were rectus at the time of initial evaluation. Eleven of the 13 feet that were not fused eventually developed a valgus deformity or severe erosions in a time period ranging from 6 to 36 months. The authors concluded that procedures not aimed at the fusion of the first MP joint will inevitably proceed to failure.

Silicone implant arthroplasty is recognized as an option in the literature. Multiple investigators have reported on the effectiveness of the double-stemmed silicone implants with and without the use of grommets in studies including patients with RA. Swanson and colleagues[8] reported on 66 feet in patients with RA who underwent implant arthroplasty, with only 3 complications noted. Two of the complications were associated with poor bone stock, resulting in rotation of the grommets. Delayed wound healing was reported only in 1 patient, which led to infection and removal of the implant. Moeckel and colleagues[9] studied 45 patients with 65 implant arthroplasties with excision of the lesser metatarsal heads. One complication was the fracture of the implant with dislocation of the joint, and 2 were postoperative infections. Cracchiolo and colleagues[10] also reported on subjective data from 86 implants (49 in patients with RA) and a nearly 7-year follow-up. At final follow-up, 8% to 4% of the patients were completely satisfied, 13% somewhat satisfied, and 3% dissatisfied. There were 2 implant failures in patients with RA and 2 failures in patients without RA. One patient with RA underwent arthrodesis after deep infection that required removal of the implant. Because of the unpredictability and increased need for secondary surgery, first MP joint arthroplasty with implant is not the preferred method of treatment for the authors of this article.

COMPLICATIONS IN HINDFOOT SURGERY

The hindfoot is affected in RA with an incidence of approximately 60% to 72%, with most degeneration beginning at the talonavicular joint, which often leads to posterior tibial tendon insufficiency, a valgus heel, and a painful rigid flatfoot.[4] Triple arthrodesis is a reasonable operative approach to this deformity assuming attempts at shoe modification and orthoses have failed.

In 2008, Knupp and colleagues[2] reported long-term results of 32 triple arthrodeses in 28 patients. Follow-up averaged 5.2 years. Complications consisted of superficial wound healing delays in 8 patients with no failed fusions. Progression of arthritis was noted in 17 cases and consisted mainly of midfoot degeneration. All patients were satisfied with the results stating that they would have the procedure again, if necessary.

Feiwell and Cracchiolo[28] reported on 16 patients (18 feet) with RA undergoing triple arthrodesis using cancellous screws for rigid fixation. Five complications were noted. Three cases of nonunion, 1 case of avascular necrosis of the talus, and 1 rocker bottom deformity in a revision case occurred. Eight of the patients with RA had continuing ankle joint degeneration, of whom 2 went on to pantalar fusion. One case of naviculocuneiform arthritis was reported.

Jones and Nunley[29] reported cases of osteonecrosis of the talar dome after triple arthrodesis in 3 patients with RA who were taking corticosteroids. In all 3 cases, the subtalar joint was fused via a dorsal-to-plantar screw orientation, which may have contributed to this complication.

COMPLICATIONS IN ANKLE AND TIBIOTALOCALCANEAL ARTHRODESIS

Pain and functional limitation in the ankle alone and the hindfoot and ankle together are also common in patients with RA. Ankle or tibiotalocalcaneal arthrodeses are procedures that offer pain relief to those suffering from the most severe manifestations of the disease in the lower extremities. Although total ankle replacement is becoming more commonplace today, ankle arthrodesis remains the gold standard with the most predictable outcomes, with fusion rates of 80% to 90%.[30] According to Mäenpää and colleagues,[30] the most common causes of failed ankle fusion are error in operative technique and failure of the surgeon to note preoperative alignment, ligamentous structural anomalies, and muscle imbalances, which should be corrected in conjunction with the arthrodesis procedure.

Felix and Kitaoka[31] studied the results of 26 ankle or tibiotalocalcaneal arthrodeses in 21 patients with RA. Ankle arthrodesis was performed in 14 ankles and tibiotalocalcaneal arthrodesis in 12. Twenty-four of the 26 were available for long-term follow-up at an average of 5 years. Union rate was 96% with only 1 nonunion, a patient who had a severe valgus hindfoot preoperatively. Delayed wound healing was noted in 2 patients who went on to complete healing uneventfully. One case of medial malleolar ulceration, 1 sural neuritis (which resolved completely), and 1 stress fracture of the tibia were also reported. The complication rate in this study was much lower than many other similar studies.

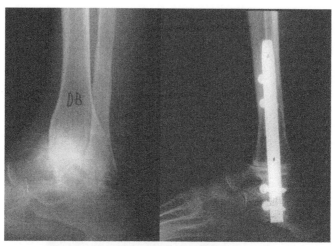

Fig. 6. Pre- and postoperative realignment of the hindfoot.

Cracchiolo and colleagues[32] reviewed 32 ankle arthrodeses in 26 patients with RA. The incidence of nonunion in these patients was 22%, infection rate 33%, malalignment 16%, and neuropraxia 9%. Moran and colleagues[33] reviewed 30 ankle arthrodeses and noted high morbidity. Forty percent of the fusions resulted in delayed wound healing, and 40% went on to nonunion. Smith and Wood[34] studied 11 ankle arthrodeses using external fixation techniques. Four patients (36%) suffered pin-tract infections, and 3 showed delayed union. All patients eventually did go on to solid union without revisional surgery. Turan and colleagues[35] reported 100% fusion of 10 ankles in 8 patients with RA, using ankle arthroscopy to assist in fusion. Subtalar joint fusion was performed in conjunction with ankle arthrodesis in 6 of the 10 feet with uneventful union. No other complications were reported in this study. Miehlke and colleagues[36] reported on 57 fusions in 43 patients (41 patients with RA) undergoing ankle, tibiotalocalcaneal, or pantalar arthrodesis. Four nonunions (7%), 2 neuropraxias (3.5%), and 2 pressure ulcers (3.5%) were reported.

Reconstruction of the hindfoot and ankle in a patient with severe deformity is a challenging task, and a systemic approach to realignment is essential. Preoperative and intraoperative radiographs should be analyzed to ensure reestablishment of the

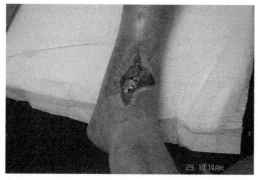

Fig. 7. Exposed total ankle replacement hardware after deep infection.

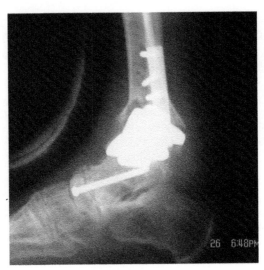

Fig. 8. Tibial fracture after component failure.

hindfoot-to-lower-leg and hindfoot-to-forefoot anatomic relationships.[37] **Fig. 6** demonstrates this principle pre- and postoperatively.

COMPLICATIONS IN TOTAL ANKLE REPLACEMENT

Because of the degeneration of proximal and distal joints after fusion, many attempts have been made to perfect ankle replacement. This would not only provide pain relief but also preserve ankle joint range of motion and slow the progression of the destruction of the joint of the midfoot. The complication rates of total ankle replacement remain higher than those of hip and total knee replacement.[32] Complications mainly surround the loosening of the implants, but occasionally, deep infections with visible components are reported (**Fig. 7**). Fracture of the tibia adjacent to the tibial component of the implant may also occur (**Fig. 8**).

Hurowitz and colleagues[38] performed a retrospective case review of 65 Agility total ankle replacements, 10 of which were performed in patients with RA. All 10 patients had successful implant outcomes at 3-year follow-up compared with 68% for post-traumatic arthritis, 42% for osteoarthritis, and 33% for nonarthritic end-stage disease (ie, adult club foot and post polio). Only one of the patients with RA in the study experienced any wound healing issues, a minor superficial wound.

Su and colleagues[39] studied second generation implants in patients with RA to compare their results with the earlier implants, which they state had reported loosening rates as high as 75% in the literature. In their study of 26 implants, 88.5% were stable at an average follow-up of 6.3 years. Complications included 1 deep infection requiring intravenous antibiotics and debridement and 1 superficial wound dehiscence that healed uneventfully with local wound care.

Kofoed and Lundberg-Jensen[40] reported on 100 total ankle replacements in 61 patients with osteoarthritis and 39 with RA. Of the patients with RA, there were 5 failed implants out of the 27 ankles available at long-term follow-up (18%). One deep infection was reported and was the cause of 1 of the 5 failed implants.

SUMMARY

Patients with RA will undoubtedly suffer from manifestations of the disease in the foot and ankle, and surgical treatment will be necessary in many cases. Although complications are inevitable in these patients, they can be minimized. Proper preoperative evaluation is a necessity. A thorough vascular examination can provide abundant information regarding healing potential. When necessary, a vascular specialist should be involved in this crucial part of the patient's care. Further complications may be prevented by maintaining a close relationship with the patient's rheumatologist regarding continuation of current medications throughout the perioperative course. Intraoperatively, careful attention should be given to anatomic and surgical principles. This includes gentle soft tissue handling, anatomic dissection, and proper realignment of bony deformities. Ample rigid fixation, whether internal or external, should always be used to provide a stable construct on which healing of fusion sites and the soft tissue envelope will occur. Postoperative management must be performed in a diligent manner, with a high suspicion for complications. When complications arise, quick and concise measures should be taken to manage them. This may include rapid use of antibiotics, surgical debridement of wounds, or revisional surgery in many cases. The combined efforts of the surgeon and supporting physicians to maintain optimal health for the patient, along with the principles previously discussed, can lead to superior outcomes with fewer complications in the postoperative course.

REFERENCES

1. Molloy AP, Myerson MS. Surgery of the lesser toes in rheumatoid arthritis: metatarsal head resection. Foot Ankle Clin 2007;12:417–33.
2. Knupp M, Skoog A, Törnkvist H, et al. Triple arthrodesis in rheumatoid arthritis. Foot Ankle Int 2008;29(3):293–7.
3. Jeng C, Campbell J. Current concepts review: the rheumatoid forefoot. Foot Ankle Int 2008;29(9):959–68.
4. Nassar J, Cracchiolo A. Complications in surgery of the foot and ankle in patients with rheumatoid arthritis. Clin Orthop Relat Res 2001;391:140–52.
5. Hansen ST Jr. The ankle and foot. In: Kelley W, Harris E, Ruddy S, et al, editors. Textbook of rheumatology. 5th edition. Philadelphia: WB Saunders; 1997. p. 1759–72.
6. Bridges SL, Moreland LW. Perioperative use of methotrexate in patients with rheumatoid arthritis undergoing orthopedic surgery. Rheum Dis Clin North Am 1997;4: 981–93.
7. Bibbo C, Anderson R, Davis W, et al. The influence of rheumatoid chemotherapy, age, and presence of rheumatoid nodules on postoperative complications in rheumatoid foot and ankle surgery: analysis of 725 procedures in 104 patients. Foot Ankle Int 2003;24(1):40–4.
8. Swanson AB, Swanson GD, Maupin BK, et al. The use of a grommet bone liner for the flexible hinge implant arthroplasty of the great toe. Foot Ankle 1991;12: 149–55.
9. Moeckel BH, Sculco TP, Alexiades MM, et al. The double-stemmed silicone-rubber implant for rheumatoid arthritis of the first metatarsophalangeal joint. Long-term results. J Bone Joint Surg Am 1992;74:564–70.
10. Cracchiolo A, Weltmer J, Lian G, et al. Arthroplasty of the first metatarsophalangeal joint with a double-stem silicone implant. J Bone Joint Surg 1992;74A: 552–63.

11. Reize P, Ina Leichtle C, Leichtle U, et al. Long-term results after metatarsal head resection in the treatment of rheumatoid arthritis. Foot Ankle Int 2006;27:586–90.

12. Anderson T, Linder L, Rydholm U, et al. Tibio-talocalcaneal arthrodesis as a primary procedure using retrograde intramedullary nail: a retrospective study of 26 patients with rheumatoid arthritis. Acta Orthop 2005;76:580–7.

13. Nagashima M, Tachihara A, Matsuzaki T, et al. Follow-up of ankle arthrodesis in severe hind foot deformity in patients with rheumatoid arthritis using an intramedullary nail with fins. Mod Rheumatol 2005;76:580–7.

14. Bibbo C. Wound healing complications and infection following surgery for rheumatoid arthritis. Foot Ankle Clin 2007;12:509–24.

15. Broeder A, Creemers M, Fransen J, et al. Risk factors for surgical site infections and other complications in elective surgery in patients with rheumatoid arthritis with special attention for anti-tumor necrosis factor: a large retrospective study. J Rheumatol 2007;34(4):689–94.

16. Grennan D, Gray J, Loudon J, et al. Methotrexate and early postoperative complications in patients with rheumatoid arthritis undergoing elective orthopaedic surgery. Ann Rheum Dis 2001;60:214–7.

17. Bibbo C, Anderson A, Davis W, et al. Rheumatoid nodules and postoperative complications. Foot Ankle Int 2003;24(1):40–4.

18. Bibbo C, Goldberg J. Infectious and healing complications after elective orthopaedic foot and ankle surgery during tumor necrosis factor-alpha inhibition therapy. Foot Ankle Int 2004;25(5):331–5.

19. Bibbo C. The assessment and perioperative management of patients with rheumatoid arthritis. Techniques Foot Ankle Surgery 2004;3:126–35.

20. Lindequw B, Rutigliano J, Williams A, et al. Prevalence of methicillin-resistant *Staphylococcus aureus* among orthopedic patients at a large academic hospital. Orthopedics 2008;31(4):363.

21. Thordarson D, Soheil A, Krieger L. Failure of hallux MP preservation surgery for rheumatoid arthritis. Foot Ankle Int 2002;23(6):486–90.

22. McGarvey SR, Johnson KA. Keller arthroplasty in combination with resection arthroplasty of the lesser metatarsophalangeal joints in rheumatoid arthrits. Foot Ankle 1988;9:75–80.

23. Cavanagh P, Ulbrecht J, Caputo G. Elevated plantar pressure and ulceration in diabetic patients after panmetatarsal head resection: two case reports. Foot Ankle Int 1999;20(8):521–6.

24. Coughlin M. Rheumatoid forefoot reconstruction. J Bone Joint Surg 2000;82:322–41.

25. Smith R, Joanis T, Maxwell P. Great toe metatarsophalangeal joint arthrodesis: a user-friendly technique. Foot Ankle 1992;13:367–77.

26. Mann R, Thompson F. Arthrodesis of the first metatarsophalangeal joint for hallux valgus in rheumatoid arthritis. J Bone Joint Surg 1984;66:687–92.

27. Mann R, Thompson F. Arthrodesis of the first metatarsophalangeal joint for hallux valgus in rheumatoid arthritis. Foot Ankle Int 1997;18(2):65–7.

28. Feiwell L, Cracchiolo A. The use of internal fixation in performing triple arthrodesis in adults. Foot 1994;4:10–4.

29. Jones C, Nunley J. Osteonecrosis of the lateral aspect of the talar dome after triple arthrodesis. J Bone Joint Surg 1999;81:1165–9.

30. Mäenpää H, Lehto M, Belt E. Why do ankle arthrodeses fail in patients with rheumatic disease? Foot Ankle Int 2001;22(5):403–8.

31. Felix N, Kitaoka H. Ankle arthrodesis in patients with rheumatoid arthritis. Clin Orthop Relat Res 1998;349:58–64.

32. Cracchiolo A, Cimina W, Lian G. Arthrodesis of the ankle in patients who have rheumatoid arthritis. J Bone Joint Surg 1992;74:903–9.
33. Moran C, Pinder I, Smith S. Ankle arthrodesis in rheumatoid arthritis. Acta Orthop Scand 1991;62:538–43.
34. Smith E, Wood P. Ankle arthrodesis in the rheumatoid patient. Foot Ankle 1990;10: 252–6.
35. Turan I, Wredmark T, Fellander-Tsia L. Arthroscopic ankle arthrodesis in rheumatoid arthritis. Clin Orthop 1995;320:110–4.
36. Miehlke W, Gschwend N, Rippstein P, et al. Compression arthrodesis of the rheumatoid ankle and hindfoot. Clin Orthop 1997;340:75–86.
37. Mendicino RW, Catanzariti AR, Reeves CL, et al. A systematic approach to evaluation of the rearfoot, ankle, and leg in reconstructive surgery. J Am Podiatr Med Assoc 2005;95(1):2–12.
38. Hurowitz E, Gould J, Fleisig G, et al. Outcome analysis of the agility total ankle replacement with prior adjunctive procedures: two to six year followup. Foot Ankle Int 2007;28(3):308–12.
39. Su E, Kahn B, Figgie M. Total ankle replacement in patients with rheumatoid arthritis. Clin Orthop Relat Res 2004;424:32–8.
40. Kofoed H, Lundberg-Jensen A. Ankle arthroplasty in patients younger and older than 50 years: a prospective series with long-term follow-up. Foot Ankle Int 1999; 20:501–6.

Subtalar Joint Arthrodesis, Ankle Arthrodiastasis, and Talar Dome Resurfacing with the Use of a Collagen-Glycosaminoglycan Monolayer

Crystal L. Ramanujam, DPM, Bryan Sagray, DPM,
Thomas Zgonis, DPM, FACFAS*

KEYWORDS

- Calcaneal fractures • Subtalar joint
- Collagen-glycosaminoglycan monolayer
- Ankle arthrodiastasis • External fixation • Ilizarov

Calcaneal fractures are a common injury to the hindfoot complex, representing 3% of all fractures and 60% of all tarsal fractures.[1,2] Essex-Lopresti[3] and Rowe and colleagues[4] reported that intraarticular injuries were present in 75% and 56% of calcaneal fractures, respectively. Typical injury patterns are a result of direct axial forces or crush trauma, seen with falls from heights and motor vehicle collisions.[1,3–6] The most common mechanism is usually from a high-energy injury involving an axial load across the ankle and subtalar joints. Concomitant fractures at sites near to or distant from the lower extremity are possible as a result of the high forces transmitted through the body during these injuries. Common sites for other osseous injuries include spinal, ankle, femoral, and wrist fractures.[7–9] In addition, transchondral injuries to the ankle joint can be sustained from a high axial load across the ankle joint and can often be missed at the time of injury.[3–9]

Division of Podiatric Medicine and Surgery, Department of Orthopaedic Surgery, The University of Texas Health Science Center at San Antonio, 7703 Floyd Curl Drive – MSC 7776, San Antonio, TX 78229, USA
* Corresponding author.
E-mail address: zgonis@uthscsa.edu

Clin Podiatr Med Surg 27 (2010) 327–333
doi:10.1016/j.cpm.2009.12.004
0891-8422/10/$ – see front matter © 2010 Elsevier Inc. All rights reserved.

podiatric.theclinics.com

Open reduction and internal fixation is currently the most widely accepted option for surgically managed calcaneal fractures.[10–15] With the advent of refined fixation and surgical techniques along with improved calcaneal plate designs, primarily those that are lower profile, complication rates have decreased. Transchondral talar dome fractures may be neglected at initial presentation, and resultant ankle joint arthrosis with restricted motion may develop. The authors describe an innovative technique of a delayed subtalar joint arthrodesis with ankle joint arthrodiastasis and talar dome resurfacing, using circular external fixation and collagen-glycosaminoglycan monolayer for a malunited calcaneal fracture with painful, restricted subtalar and ankle joint motion.

CASE REPORT

A 48-year-old male presented to the clinic complaining of persistent pain and difficulty with ambulation after previous percutaneous screw fixation of a calcaneal fracture to the left foot. He had suffered a 10-ft fall from a ladder, approximately 2 years earlier. He sustained no other injuries at the time and reported having been treated surgically within the first few days of the fall. The patient's past medical history was significant for diabetes mellitus, hyperlipidemia, and depression. Previous surgeries included back surgery and left ankle surgery as a child. He admitted to smoking a pack of cigarettes every other day for 20 years. Before the calcaneal fracture, the patient had maintained an active lifestyle and worked as a maintenance repairman.

Lower extremity physical examination revealed mild nonpitting edema to the left ankle and rearfoot. Sensation was grossly intact and muscle strength was normal. Most notably there was pain on palpation to the sinus tarsi, lateral ankle gutter, deltoid ligament, and collateral ligaments. Restricted and painful motion was noted in the subtalar and ankle joints.

Foot, ankle, and calcaneal axial weight-bearing radiographs demonstrated retained hardware at the left calcaneus. Evidence of left subtalar joint arthrosis was noted compared with the contralateral foot, as well as decreased joint space at the ankle joint with mild sclerosis on the adjacent talar dome, suspicious for a previous transchondral fracture. The left foot also revealed varus malunion of the calcaneus with decreased talar declination from residual posterior facet depression. There was no apparent anterior ankle joint impingement or calcaneocuboid joint arthrosis. Computed tomography confirmed extensive arthrosis to the subtalar joint with moderate involvement of the ankle.

Based on all findings, conservative and surgical options were discussed with the patient and he elected to proceed with surgical intervention. The goals of surgical care were to decrease pain and preserve ankle joint range of motion. Informed consent was obtained for removal of hardware, subtalar joint arthrodesis with internal fixation, open ankle arthrotomy with resurfacing of the talus using a collagen-glycosaminoglycan monolayer, and ankle arthrodiastasis with circular external fixation.

The patient was taken to the operating room and placed under general anesthesia with endotracheal intubation. He was prepped and draped in the usual sterile fashion and a sterile thigh tourniquet was placed on the left lower extremity inflated to 350 mm Hg. A bump of towels was placed under the ipsilateral hip to facilitate internal rotation of the lower extremity and the leg was draped above the knee to allow visualization of the patella and axial alignment of the leg during surgery.

The existing hardware was removed through a trans-Achilles approach and a bone anchor was used to reattach the distal aspect of the Achilles tendon. A lateral extensile incision was then made, modified by performing the horizontal limb in a lazy "S" fashion. The modification was designed to allow distraction bone block arthrodesis of the subtalar joint if necessary or concomitant ankle arthrodiastasis without concern for tension on the skin edges because of increased limb length.[16] The subtalar joint was identified and prepared for in situ fusion by removal of cartilage at the talar and calcaneal surfaces in addition to subchondral drilling to an adequate level to reveal bleeding, healthy bone. Demineralized bone matrix allograft was packed into the freshly prepared joint space. Under fluoroscopic guidance, a single 7.5-mm partially short-threaded cannulated cancellous screw was placed across the joint with correction of varus deformity and adequate compression observed. The lateral incision was carefully closed in layered fashion. Next, an anterior ankle arthrotomy was performed to expose the ankle joint. Hypertrophied, inflamed synovium and a small tibial exostosis were debrided to relieve impingement. Visualized transchondral lesions were also addressed by using the microfracture technique.[17] A 2 × 2-in single collagen-glycosaminoglycan monolayer (Integra Lifesciences, Plainsboro, NJ, USA) was then placed over the entire surface of the talar dome followed by fibrin sealant application **(Fig. 1)**. The inflated tourniquet was released after skin closure and before the application of the circular external fixation frame.

The prebuilt circular external fixation frame was positioned on the foot and lower extremity. Frontal plane wires followed by oblique plane wires were then inserted into the calcaneus, proximal tibia, and distal tibia. These 1.8-mm wires were secured to the circular external fixation frame and tensioned by a mechanical tensioner in

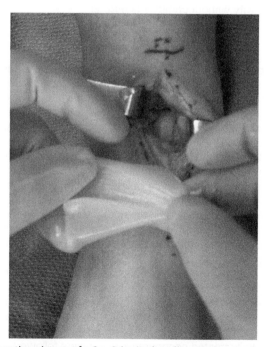

Fig. 1. An intraoperative picture of a 2 × 2-in single collagen-glycosaminoglycan monolayer (Integra Lifesciences, Plainsboro, NJ, USA) for talar resurfacing at the ankle joint. A fibrin sealant is used to allow incorporation and minimize graft movement. This is a different case demonstrating the technique and unrelated to **Fig. 2**.

a standard manner. A talar wire was also placed and secured to the foot plate before the ankle distraction technique was performed. Next, the threaded rods that connected the foot plate to the distal tibia ring were loosened, allowing for 10 mm of acute ankle joint distraction. At this point the ankle was distracted and the threaded rods were tightened. An additional fine wire was placed across the midfoot to prevent an equinus contracture and to reduce torsional forces from the foot. This 10-mm distance was determined to allow the subchondral bone to be off-loaded without risk of acute neurovascular compromise. A large, bulky sterile dressing was applied to the construct to prevent movement of the wires at the dermal interface.[17–20]

Postoperatively, the patient was admitted to the hospital for observation, deep vein thrombosis prophylaxis, antibiotics, pain management, and physical therapy for non–weight bearing to the left foot. Once the patient's pain level and ambulatory status were adequately addressed, the patient was discharged from the hospital. The patient was followed up in the outpatient setting at 2-week intervals for incision and wire site care, and serial radiographs were taken to evaluate for subtalar joint consolidation, alignment, and maintenance of the ankle joint arthrodiastasis. Once complete consolidation at the subtalar joint was observed by radiographic parameters, the circular external fixation frame was removed. The patient was progressed to a non–weight bearing, fiberglass, short leg cast for 3 weeks, followed by full weight bearing in a removable surgical boot for 8 weeks, and then finally transitioned into regular footwear.

Ultimately, complete fusion of the subtalar joint was achieved with correction of the varus hindfoot deformity. At 8 months' follow-up, the patient reported pain-free motion at the ankle joint complex with adequate dorsiflexion observed. He returned to work and recreational activity without complaints (**Fig. 2**).

DISCUSSION

Residual hindfoot deformities and posttraumatic arthrosis can occur after intraarticular calcaneal fractures.[21–23] The presentation of a varus malunited calcaneal fracture with posterior facet depression and concomitant subtalar and ankle joint arthrosis is challenging for any treating surgeon. Surgeons frequently use a stepwise approach to deformity correction with hindfoot arthrodesis and calcaneal osteotomies as mainstay therapies.

Stephens and Sanders[15] devised a classification system with an accompanying treatment algorithm for malunited calcaneal fractures. Their system divided the fractures into types based on the presence of lateral wall exostosis, degree of subtalar joint arthrosis, and presence of varus/valgus angulation. The combination and severity of these parameters found on computed tomography determined the class of the malunion and reconstructive approach used to achieve resolution. Treatment progressed from lateral wall ostectomy, partial subtalar joint resection and early mobilization, to subtalar joint arthrodesis and calcaneal osteotomies corresponding to each type. Although some of their original patients had calcaneocuboid joint involvement, no patients required triple arthrodesis once treatment was carried out.

Recently, a study by Randay and colleagues[24] found that patients with calcaneal fractures had much better functional outcomes through initial open reduction with internal fixation and delayed subtalar joint arthrodesis if necessary. Residual malunions that were initially treated nonoperatively and were followed by delayed reconstruction had more postoperative wound complications and functional impairment. These findings stress the importance of proper fracture reduction on initial presentation to restore the anatomic shape and articular congruity of the calcaneus.

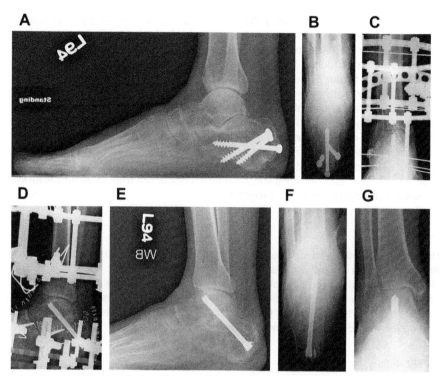

Fig. 2. Preoperative lateral (*A*) and calcaneal axial (*B*) radiographic views showing prominent hardware in addition to the decreased and arthritic space at the subtalar and ankle joints. Postoperative anteroposterior (*C*) and lateral (*D*) ankle views showing the ankle arthrodiastasis using the circular external fixation frame and subtalar joint arthrodesis with internal fixation. The patient also had a talar resurfacing procedure using a single collagen-glycosaminoglycan monolayer (Integra Lifesciences, Plainsboro, NJ, USA). The circular external fixation system was removed at 7 weeks postoperatively. Final postoperative lateral (*E*), calcaneal axial (*F*) and ankle anteroposterior (*G*) radiographic views at 8 months follow-up.

The development of ankle arthrosis as a result of a severe intraarticular calcaneal fracture may be rare but should be addressed when present, especially if a subtalar joint arthrodesis is required. After subtalar joint arthrodesis, compensatory motion and stress will be encountered at the ankle and midfoot joints, resulting in exacerbation and progression of any preexisting symptoms and joint degeneration.

In the correct patient population, hindfoot arthrodesis combined with ankle arthroplasty or arthrodiastasis can be a sound adjuvant.[20] An isolated arthrodesis of the subtalar joint is well tolerated in the young active patient with slight activity modification. If concomitant ankle joint and subtalar joint arthrodesis is performed, activity becomes much more limited and alternate options such as ankle arthrodiastasis become more applicable.

Arthrodiastasis facilitates intermittent increases in joint pressures within the ankle joint while offloading the joint surfaces.[18] These changes in joint pressure are thought to cause a corresponding increase in proteoglycan synthesis which, in the absence of mechanical stress, promotes cartilage repair.[25] Judet and Judet[26] first described arthrodiastasis in a canine model; they observed normal articular cartilage repair within a year. Aldegheri and colleagues[27] later demonstrated this procedure for the treatment of hip arthritis; their results were good in 71% of patients under 45 years of age. Van Valburg and colleagues[28] first reported on ankle arthrodiastasis using circular external fixation to delay the need for ankle arthrodesis. Many authors also advocate arthroscopic debridement, loose-body removal, cheilectomy, and/or microfracture at the time of external fixator placement.[18]

Open ankle arthrotomy provides better access to the joint interfaces for treatment and facilitates the placement of the collagen-glycosaminoglycan monolayer to the talar dome if needed.[20,23] It is hypothesized that placement of the acellular monolayer graft, along with microfracture technique of talar transchondral injuries, promotes neovascularization and cellular repopulation for repair of the joint surface.[29] Overall bone loss with our combination of procedures is minimal, leaving more aggressive surgical treatment options, such as ankle implant arthroplasty or arthrodesis, available for later use should the disease process progress.

SUMMARY

The technique of delayed subtalar joint arthrodesis, ankle joint arthrodiastasis, and talar resurfacing is a new approach to managing posttraumatic subtalar and ankle arthrosis. The authors remain optimistic that this will become a reproducible and reliable means of treating this condition especially amongst the younger population. The surgeon must be familiar with all the necessary techniques, as these procedures have a steep learning curve and require surgical experience.

REFERENCES

1. Cave EF. Fracture of the os calcis – the problem in general. Clin Orthop Relat Res 1963;30:64–6.
2. Eastwood WJ. Fracture of the os calcis. Br J Surg 1938;25:636–46.
3. Essex-Lopresti P. The mechanism, reduction technique, and results in fractures of the os calcis. Br J Surg 1952;39:395–419.
4. Rowe CR, Sakellarides H, Freeman P. Fractures of os calcis – a long term follow-up study of one hundred forty-six patients. JAMA 1963;184:920–3.
5. Crosby LA, Kamins P. The history of the calcaneal fracture. Orthop Rev 1991;20: 501–9.
6. Warrick CK, Borrelli J, Lashgari, et al. Fractures of the calcaneum – with an atlas illustrating the various types of fracture. J Bone Joint Surg Br 1954;35:33–4.
7. Wong PN. Vertebral column and os calcis fracture patterns in a confined community (Singapore). Acta Orthop Scand 1966;37:357–66.
8. Lance EM, Carey EJ, Wade PA. Fractures of the os calcis – a follow-up study. J Trauma 1964;4:15–46.
9. Chou LB, Lee DC. Current concept review: perioperative soft tissue management for foot and ankle fractures. Foot Ankle Int 2009;30(1):84–90.
10. Sanders R. Displaced intra-articular fractures of the calcaneus. J Bone Joint Surg Am 2000;82(2):225–50.
11. McGarvey WC, Burris MW, Clanton TO, et al. Calcaneal fractures: indirect reduction and external fixation. Foot Ankle Int 2006;27(7):494–9.
12. Weber M, Lehmann O, Sagesser D, et al. Limited open reduction and internal fixation of displaced intra-articular fractures of the calcaneum. J Bone Joint Surg Br 2007;90(12):1608–16.
13. Stulik J, Stehlik J, Rysavy M, et al. Minimally-invasive treatment of intra-articular fracture of the calcaneum. J Bone Joint Surg Br 2005;88(12):1634–41.

14. Clare MP, Lee WE, Sanders RW. Intermediate to long-term results of a treatment protocol for calcaneal fracture malunion. J Bone Joint Surg Am 2005;87(5): 963–73.
15. Stephens HM, Sanders R. Calcaneal malunions: results of a prognostic computed tomography classification system. Foot Ankle Int 1996;17(7):395–401.
16. Garras DN, Santangelo JR, Wang DW, et al. Subtalar distraction arthrodesis using interpositional frozen structural allograft. Foot Ankle Int 2008;29(6):561–7.
17. Morse KR, Flemister AS, Baumhauer JF, et al. Distraction arthroplasty. Foot Ankle Clin 2007;12(1):29–39.
18. Martin RL, Stewart GW, Conti SF. Posttraumatic ankle arthritis: an update on conservative and surgical management. J Orthop Sports Phys Ther 2007;37(5): 253–9.
19. Paley D, Lamm BM, Purohit RM, et al. Distraction arthroplasty of the ankle – how far can you stretch the indications? Foot Ankle Clin 2008;13(3):471–84.
20. Zgonis T, Stapleton JJ, Roukis TS. Use of circular external fixation for combined subtalar joint arthrodesis and ankle distraction. Clin Podiatr Med Surg 2008;25(4): 745–53.
21. Reddy V, Fukuda T, Ptaszek AJ. Calcaneus malunion and nonunion. Foot Ankle Clin 2007;12(1):125–35.
22. Anderson LB, Stauff MP, Juliano PJ. Combined subtalar and ankle arthritis. Foot Ankle Clin 2007;12:57–73.
23. Stapleton JJ, Belczyk R, Zgonis T. Surgical treatment of calcaneal fracture malunion and posttraumatic deformities. Clin Podiatr Med Surg 2009;26(1):79–90.
24. Randay CS, Clare MP, Sanders RW. Subtalar fusion after displaced intra-articular calcaneal fractures: does initial operative treatment matter. J Bone Joint Surg Am 2009;91(3):541–6.
25. Lafeber F, Veldhuijzen JP, Vanroy JL, et al. Intermittent hydrostatic compressive force stimulates exclusively the proteoglycan synthesis of osteoarthritic human cartilage. Br J Rheumatol 1992;31(7):437–42.
26. Judet R, Judet T. The use of a hinge distraction apparatus after arthrolysis and arthroplasty. Rev Chir Orthop Reparatrice Appar Mot 1978;64(5):353–65.
27. Aldegheri R, Trivella G, Saleh M. Articulated distraction of the hip. Conservative surgery for arthritis in young patients. Clin Orthop Relat Res 1994;301:94–101.
28. Van Valburg AA, van Roermund PM, Lammens J, et al. Can Ilizarov joint distraction delay the need for an arthrodesis of the ankle? A preliminary report. J Bone Joint Surg Br 1995;77(5):720–5.
29. Berlet GC, Hyer CF, Lee TH, et al. Interpositional arthroplasty of the first MTP joint using a regenerative tissue matrix for the treatment of advanced hallux rigidus. Foot Ankle Int 2008;29(1):10–21.

Selective Percutaneous Myofascial Lengthening of the Lower Extremities in Children with Spastic Cerebral Palsy

Evanthia A. Mitsiokapa, MD[a], Andreas F. Mavrogenis, MD[b],
Helen Skouteli, MD[c], Stamatios G. Vrettos, MS[d],
George Tzanos, MD, DSc[a], Anastasios D. Kanellopoulos, MD, DSc[b],
Demetrios S. Korres, MD[e],
Panayiotis J. Papagelopoulos, MD, DSc[b],*

KEYWORDS

- Cerebral palsy • Spasticity
- Gross motor function classification system
- Gross motor function measure
- Selective percutaneous myofascial lengthening

Cerebral palsy is a disorder of movement and posture resulting from a nonprogressive injury to the immature brain. It is one of the most common developmental disabilities. The estimated prevalence is 2.0 to 2.5 per 1000 live births, and its manifestations often progress as the child matures.[1,2] The most common movement disorder in cerebral palsy is spastic. Children with spastic cerebral palsy commonly acquire musculoskeletal deformities, including progressive joint contractures, shortened muscles, hip dysplasia, and neuromuscular scoliosis. These manifestations will, at some point need orthopaedic surgery.[3] This type of surgery, however, is associated with increased surgical trauma, length of hospital stay, and patient and family inconvenience.[4] The purpose of this retrospective study was to assess the effect of selective

[a] Department of Physical Medicine and Rehabilitation, Thriasio Hospital, 19018 Elefsina, Greece
[b] First Department of Orthopaedics, Athens University Medical School, 41 Ventouri Street, 15562 Holargos, Athens, Greece
[c] 11634 Pagkzati, Athens, Greece
[d] 15234 Halandri, Athens, Greece
[e] Third Department of Orthopaedics, Athens University Medical School, Nikis 2, 14561 Kifisia, Athens, Greece
* Corresponding author.
E-mail address: pjportho@otenet.gr

Clin Podiatr Med Surg 27 (2010) 335–343
doi:10.1016/j.cpm.2009.12.005
0891-8422/10/$ – see front matter © 2010 Elsevier Inc. All rights reserved.

podiatric.theclinics.com

percutaneous myofascial lengthening on the functional improvement of spastic cerebral palsy in children.

MATERIALS AND METHODS

A retrospective review of 58 children with spastic cerebral palsy who underwent selective percutaneous myofascial lengthening of the hip adductor group, and the medial or the lateral hamstrings was conducted at the Department of Pediatric Orthopaedic Surgery of Athens University School of Medicine from January 2003 to December 2006. There were 16 boys and 42 girls, aged 3 to 12 years. All patients were spastic diplegic, hemiplegic, or quadriplegic, and their cognition and emotional maturation were adequate to comply with postoperative rehabilitation.

The indications for surgery were primary contractures that interfered with the patients' walking or sitting ability, or joint subluxation. The primary objective of surgery was to improve the patients' level of motor function and to prevent the development of secondary contractures in the hips, knees, and ankles with the minimum compromise on patient comfort. Children with previous neurosurgical procedures such as selective dorsal rhizotomy or intrathecal baclofen, combined deformities and severe lower extremity spasticity that necessitated combined orthopedic surgical procedures were excluded.

Initial neurologic, physical medicine, and physical therapist assessment of gross motor function were completed before the procedure. Children were classified by age and gross motor ability using the gross motor function classification system (GMFCS).[5] This system reflects a child's current abilities, self-initiated movements, and limitations in gross motor function, with emphasis on function in sitting and walking. The GMFCS is not an outcome measure. It is a classification that is stable over time in 80% to 85% of children irrespective of intervention. GMFCS includes five levels based on the degree of independence and efficiency of motor function.[5,6]

Gross motor function was measured using the original 88-item gross motor function measure (GMFM-88) that was designed and validated to evaluate changes over time in children with cerebral palsy.[5,7–9] The GMFM is a standardized quantitative assessment scale of gross motor function, with good intrarater (0.92 to 0.99) and inter-rater (0.87 to 0.99) reliability that has been shown of good validity (0.66 to 0.79) to demonstrate change in function over time. The GMFM provides an assessment of an artificial performance in a controlled environment as a change in body function. It measures at best what a child can do, rather than what a child does do. The GMFM total scores can range from 0 to 100.[7,10] All children included in this study were at GMFCS levels 1 to 4, and had a mean GMFM of 71.19 points. The data of the 58 patients were collected and analyzed (Table 1).

The procedure of selective percutaneous myofascial lengthening or the percutaneous (PERCS) procedure, as described by Roy Nuzzo,[11,12] was performed under general anesthesia and without the use of muscle relaxants. This allowed for of the use of nerve stimulation to easily locate the obturator nerve and to proceed with its blockade. The procedure involved releasing the tight bands of tendon contractures (Fig. 1). This was performed at the muscolotendinous junctions and where part of the myofascia complex was found to be thickened and shortened. When the myofascia was released, the muscle could be stretched and lengthened easily. Lengthening of the musculotendinous unit decreased the spasticity in that area. Minimal surgical incisions were used, and very little scarring was formed as a result of the procedure. This is an advantage of selective percutaneous myofascial lengthening, since scar is known to be associated with recurrent contractures. In addition, it allows the procedure to work well for all ages, including groups that have a tendency for recurrent contractures following conventional tendon lengthening surgery, such as very young children and adolescents.[11,12]

Of the 58 children involved in this study, 47 had selective percutaneous myofascial lengthening of the hip adductors and the hamstrings, in addition to alcohol blockade of the obturator nerve. Two of these children had additional lengthening of the tensor fascia lata and santorius muscles. Eight hemiplegics had isolated percutaneous myofascial lengthening of the hamstrings; one of them had additional lengthening of the tensor fascia lata and santorius muscles. Three children had isolated percutaneous myofascial lengthening of the hip adductors, in addition to alcohol blockade of the obturator nerve.

A few hours after the operation, the children were discharged from the hospital setting and were allowed for same-day ambulation, bracing, and physical therapy. All families received instructions for the importance of mobility in all types of surfaces according to the functional level of each child. Bracing schemes involved the use of a solid ankle foot orthosis to control the foot and provide a sound basis for the stance phase of the gait cycle and a knee immobilizer for the first 1 to 2 weeks. Hamstring stretching exercises were instructed for 2 hours per day for 1 week, in addition to instructions for three to five sessions per week of physical therapy, and participation of families in the mobility program of their children. Postoperative assessment of the GMFCS and the GMFM was done at 6, 12, and 24 months of therapy (see **Table 1**).

RESULTS

The mean time of the surgical procedures was 14 minutes (range, 1 to 27 minutes). The surgical wounds were minor, and postoperative recovery was uneventful in all patients. There were no infections, overlengthening, nerve palsies, or vascular complications. Three patients required repeated procedures for relapsed hamstring and adductor contractures at 8, 14, and 16 months postoperatively. None of those three patients who required revisional surgery followed the postoperative bracing protocol as recommended. At 2 years postoperatively, all children improved on their previous functional level (see **Table 1**). Thirty-four children improved by one GMFCS level, and five children improved by two GMFCS levels. This finding is of functional significance, because the GMFCS is considered to be stable over time.[5,6] The overall improvement in mean GMFM scores was from 71.19 to 83.19.

DISCUSSION

The goals of management of spasticity in children with cerebral palsy are to maximize active function, ease care, and prevent secondary problems such as pain, joint subluxation, and contractures. When a management option is being considered, its impact on cost, time demands of the family, social limitations, psychological issues, and potential complications needs to be reviewed in detail. The purpose of this study was to report results on the management of children with spastic cerebral palsy of the lower extremities using selective percutaneous myofascial lengthening.

Currently, there are no meaningful interventions that can successfully repair existing damage to the brain areas that control muscle coordination and movement. Several treatments, however, including new therapeutic agents, surgical techniques, and novel physical therapy and rehabilitation regimens are available to diminish the degree of impairment from muscle spasticity and joint contractures, and to increase participation in activities of daily living.[11–16]

Table 1
The preoperative, 6-, 12-, and 24-month GMFCS and GMFM classification of the 58 children involved in this study

Patients	Presurgery		After 6 Months		After 1 Year		After 2 Years	
	GMFCS	GMFM	GMFCS	GMFM	GMFCS	GMFM	GMFCS	GMFM
1	1	92	1	96	1	98	1	98
2	1	94	1	98	1	98	1	98
3	1	95	1	98	1	98	1	98
4	2	88	1	95	1	96	1	98
5	2	82	1	88	1	94	1	96
6	2	86	1	95	1	95	1	95
7	2	85	1	96	1	96	1	96
8	2	82	1	88	1	91	1	91
9	2	76	2	84	2	87	2	89
10	2	88	1	95	1	98	1	98
11	2	88	1	95	1	98	1	98
12	2	82	2	89	1	93	1	95
13	2	78	2	87	1	91	1	93
14	2	76	2	83	2	88	2	88
15	2	86	2	95	2	95	2	95
16	2	95	1	98	1	98	1	98
17	2	72	2	84	2	86	2	87
18	2	74	2	82	2	84	2	84
19	2	79	2	87	1	94	1	94
20	2	88	2	92	1	95	1	97
21	2	78	2	85	2	86	2	88
22	3	78	2	86	2	87	2	88
23	3	78	2	85	2	85	2	88
24	3	65	3	72	2	78	2	78
25	3	80	2	86	2	88	2	91
26	3	65	3	72	3	75	3	76
27	3	80	2	92	2	95	2	95
28	3	66	2	75	2	75	2	75
29	3	76	1	84	1	88	1	88
30	3	68	2	87	2	93	1	95
31	3	69	2	78	2	82	2	85
32	3	72	2	86	2	88	1	95
33	3	74	1	86	1	92	1	92
34	3	69	2	78	2	82	2	85
35	3	64	3	72	3	72	3	72
36	3	70	3	78	3	78	3	78
37	3	68	2	79	2	79	2	84
38	3	72	2	82	2	84	2	88
39	3	72	2	85	2	88	1	95
40	3	64	3	73	3	73	3	73

(continued on next page)

Table 1
(continued)

Patients	Presurgery		After 6 Months		After 1 Year		After 2 Years	
	GMFCS	GMFM	GMFCS	GMFM	GMFCS	GMFM	GMFCS	GMFM
41	3	69	2	78	2	81	2	81
42	3	83	2	88	2	91	2	91
43	3	67	3	73	3	75	3	77
44	3	65	3	73	3	76	3	78
45	3	62	3	71	3	75	3	75
46	3	67	2	76	2	78	2	78
47	3	68	2	74	2	78	2	78
48	3	85	2	86	2	88	2	88
49	3	78	2	85	2	87	2	88
50	3	76	3	83	2	87	2	88
51	3	65	3	70	3	89	3	89
52	4	29	4	34	4	34	4	34
53	4	42	3	54	3	64	3	64
54	4	30	3	45	3	46	3	46
55	4	33	3	41	3	45	3	48
56	4	30	3	36	3	42	3	42
57	4	31	3	38	3	41	3	43
58	4	35	4	38	4	42	4	42

Abbreviations: GMFCS, gross motor function classification system; GMFM, gross motor function measure.

Oral antispasticity agents such as baclofen, tizanidine, clonazepam, diazepam, and dantrolene sodium are most appropriate for children who need only mild tone reduction or have diffuse spasticity. Despite ease of use, they are associated with significant adverse effects such as hepatotoxicity, drowsiness, muscle weakness, constipation, and sedation.[17] Upper[18] and lower extremity[19,20] intramuscular injections of botulinum toxin-A have been reported to improve function significantly and ease pain.[21] The lowest effective dose with an injection interval of at least 3 months or more should be used to minimize the risk of antibody development and immunoresistance.[16,22,23] Chemodenervation using phenol and alcohol is characterized by the absence of immunogenicity and the lower cost compared with botulinum toxin,[15,24,25] but it is associated with complications such as sensory loss and pain or paresthesias when targeting a mixed nerve, which may be permanent.[15,24]

Selective dorsal rhizotomy, although it reduces spasticity, it is a major neurosurgical operation, with increased surgical trauma, hospitalization, and cost, and it is associated with complications including back pain, sensory changes, and neurogenic bladder or bowel problems in up to 30% of patients.[26,27] Intrathecal baclofen has been shown to reduce spasticity in cerebral palsy producing some functional improvement[28,29]; however, it requires an implantable pump and transcutaneous refills every 2 to 3 months. Additionally, it is associated with serious complications such as abrupt withdrawal of the catheter and overdose from a programming error that may lead to respiratory depression, coma, and death.[15,30]

Traditional orthopedic surgical treatments for children with cerebral palsy were tendon lengthenings or transfers, bone fusions, and derotation osteotomies that

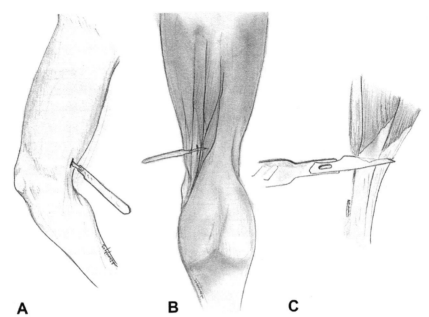

A   **B**   **C**

Fig. 1. (*A*) A small skin incision is made at the myofascial junction of a tight/spastic high-velocity muscle (a muscle with long excursion) such as the hamstrings (as illustrated), the hip adductors, the tensor fascia lata, the santorius, and the heel cord. (*B, C*) Tight bands of tendon are released percutaneously at the myofascia over the muscle surface. When the myofascia is cut, the muscle under it can stretch and lengthen easily.

were performed through an open surgical procedure.[13,31] Open surgical procedures, however, have been associated with increased complication rates, including major surgical trauma, increased length of hospital stay, hemorrhage, hematoma formation, infections, skin problems, compartment syndrome, heterotopic ossification,[32,33] tendon scarring,[15–17,34] recurrent knee flexion postures, especially in severely involved children, need of casting, and revision surgery[15,35,36] or re-operation.[13,31] In the present series, an outpatient procedure called selective percutaneous myofascial lengthening was undertaken in children up to 12 years of age with excellent results.

Selective percutaneous myofascial lengthening has the benefit of minimally invasive orthopedic surgery combined with immediate initiation of physical therapy and rehabilitation. It was initiated over 25 years ago as a make-do in children with severe cardiac conditions and serious risks for the routine orthopedic surgical interventions with the anesthesia requirements.[11,12] Lengthening initially was derived from fields of disconnected small cuts (similar to mesh skin grafting) in the myofascia over the muscle surface. Initial results were excellent, leading to generalization of its application. From the early observations, strategies evolved, including

Targeting high-velocity muscles (attachment furthest from joint center as more stimulating of spasticity)

Avoidance of same-session single joint muscles in ambulators (to preserve adaptive control mechanisms)

Avoidance of ranges of motion exceeding control capability (speed of response)

Lengthening only palpably taut portions of the selected myofascia (commonly less than 10% of the width) (Nuzzo RM, unpublished data, 2004).[11,12]

Percutaneous myofascial lengthening relates to a type of surgery applicable to cerebral palsy, chronic illness, spina bifida, congenital defects, and various other reconstructive problems. It is an approach to muscle reactivity, range, and control. It is designed with respect to the neurologic control mechanisms, and although it is involved with creating length, length is not its singular goal in most cases. The technique is based on the very same methods used by plastic surgeons to stretch small skin grafts over large burn areas, but, in children with cerebral palsy, it instead is applied to deeper structures, and only the most over-reactive subset of muscles.[11,12]

Percutaneous myofascial lengthening yields the merits of same-day rehabilitation. Physical therapy may initiate ambulation, stretching, and range-of-motion exercises from the very first postoperative day. In this current study, the authors have used a knee immobilizer for muscle stretching and an ankle foot orthosis to control the foot and provide a sound basis for ambulation. Also, percutaneous myofascial lengthening does not cause muscle weakness, muscle contractures, significant pain, or scar tissue formation around the soft tissue. Minimal scarring allows the surgeon to offer this type of procedure in younger patients, because the condition of the soft tissues is not altered, thus allowing repeated procedures if required.

Following surgical intervention, early institution of a physical therapy and rehabilitation program and home stretching excercises is essential for children with cerebral palsy to keep spastic muscles stretched, improve muscle strength and coordination, optimize muscle length, maintain range of motion, diminish disability, improve function, and maintain performance in meaningful tasks.[16,17]

SUMMARY

The management of spasticity in children with cerebral palsy is complex and best provided in a multidisciplinary team approach with input from physical therapists and pedorthitists. Selective percutaneous myofascial lengthening enhanced by same-day initiation of physical therapy and rehabilitation is a safe, minimally invasive outpatient procedure with excellent results in spastic children. Finally, the authors believe that a longer follow-up period, during which most of the patients reach skeletal maturity, is crucial to demonstrate the effectiveness of this treatment and to validate the protocol used.

ACKNOWLEDGMENTS

The authors wish to thank Dimitris Antonopoulos, MD, for the medical illustrations of the technique presented in this article.

REFERENCES

1. Nelson KB, Grether JK. Causes of cerebral palsy. Curr Opin Pediatr 1999;11: 487–91.
2. Nelson K. Can we prevent cerebral palsy? N Engl J Med 2003;349:1765–9.
3. DeLuca PA. The musculoskeletal management of children with cerebral palsy. Pediatr Clin North Am 1996;43:1135–50.
4. Murphy NA, Hoff C, Jorgensen T, et al. Costs and complications of hospitalizations for children with cerebral palsy. Pediatr Rehabil 2006;9(1):47–52.
5. Palisano R, Rosenbaum P, Walter S, et al. Development and reliability of a system to classify gross motor function in children with cerebral palsy. Dev Med Child Neurol 1997;39(4):214–23.

6. Rosenbaum PL, Walter SD, Hanna SE, et al. Prognosis for gross motor function in cerebral palsy. Creation of motor development curves. JAMA 2002;288:1357–63.

7. Russell DJ, Rosenbaum PL, Cadman DT, et al. The gross motor function measure: a means to evaluate the effects of physical therapy. Dev Med Child Neurol 1989; 31(3):341–52.

8. Russell D, Rosenbaum P, Gowland C, et al. Gross motor function measure manual. 2nd edititon. Hamilton (Ontario, Canada): McMaster University; 1993.

9. Russell D, Avery L, Rosenbaum P, et al. Improved scaling of the gross motor function measure for children with cerebral palsy: evidence of reliability and validity. Phys Ther 2000;80(9):873–85.

10. Palisano RJ, Hanna SE, Rosenbaum PL, et al. Validation of a model of gross motor function for children with cerebral palsy. Phys Ther 2000;80:974–85.

11. Nuzzo RM. SPMLs—selective percutaneous myofascial lengthening in velocity-dependant neuromuscular gamma-efferent high gain feedback oscillation syndromes—or how I came to like the word "percs". Cerebral Palsy Magazine 2004;2(4):30–7.

12. Selective percutaneous myofascial lengthening. (SPML) percutaneous muscle/tendon lengthening, SPLs, "percs," "Gucci procedure" (and other nastier names). Accessed at: http://www.pediatric-orthopedics.com/Treatments/Perc_Lengthening/perc_lengthening.html. Accessed January 3, 2010.

13. Patrick JH, Roberts AP, Cole GF. Therapeutic choices in the locomotor management of the child with cerebral palsy—more luck than judgement? Arch Dis Child 2001;85:275–9.

14. Goldstein M. The treatment of cerebral palsy: what we know, what we don't know. J Pediatr 2004;145:S42–6.

15. Tilton AH. Management of spasticity in children with cerebral palsy. Semin Pediatr Neurol 2004;11(1):58–65.

16. Steinbok P. Selection of treatment modalities in children with spastic cerebral palsy. Neurosurg Focus 2006;21(2):E4.

17. Jacobs JM. Management options for the child with spastic cerebral palsy. Orthop Nurs. 2001;20(3):53–61.

18. Fehlings D, Rang M, Glazier J, et al. An evaluation of botulinum-A toxin injections to improve upper extremity function in children with hemiplegic cerebral palsy. J Pediatr 2000;137(3):331–7.

19. Ubhi T, Bhakta BB, Ives HL, et al. Randomized double-blind placebo-controlled trial of the effect of botulinum toxin on walking in cerebral palsy. Arch Dis Child 2000;83(6):481–7.

20. Love SC, Valentine JP, Blair EM, et al. The effect of botulinum toxin type A on the functional ability of the child with spastic hemiplegia: a randomized controlled trial. Eur J Neurol 2001;8(Suppl 5):50–8.

21. Barwood S, Baillieu C, Boyd R, et al. Analgesic effects of botulinum toxin A: a randomized, placebo-controlled clinical trial. Dev Med Child Neurol 2000; 42(2):116–21.

22. Jankovic J, Vuong KD, Ahsan J. Comparison of efficacy and immunogenicity of original versus current botulinum toxin in cervical dystonia. Neurology 2003;60: 1186–8.

23. Boyd RN, Hays RM. Current evidence for the use of botulinum toxin type A in the management of children with cerebral palsy: a systematic review. Eur J Neurol 2001;8S(5):1–20.

24. Tilton AH. Injectable neuromuscular blockade in the treatment of spasticity and movement disorders. J Child Neurol 2003;18:S50–66.

25. Smyth MD, Peacock WJ. The surgical treatment of spasticity. Muscle Nerve 2000; 23:153–63.
26. Engsberg JR, Ross SA, Wagner JM, et al. Changes in hip spasticity and strength following selective dorsal rhizotomy and physical therapy for spastic cerebral palsy. Dev Med Child Neurol 2002;44(4):220–6.
27. Steinbok P, Schrag C. Complications after selective posterior rhizotomy for spasticity in children with cerebral palsy. Pediatr Neurosurg 1998;28:300–13.
28. Van Schaeybroeck P, Nuttin B, Lagae L, et al. Intrathecal baclofen for intractable cerebral spasticity: a prospective placebo-controlled, double-blind study. Neurosurgery 2003;46(3):603–12.
29. Awaad Y, Tayem H, Munoz S, et al. Functional assessment following intrathecal baclofen therapy in children with spastic cerebral palsy. J Child Neurol 2003; 18(1):26–34.
30. Coffey RJ, Edgar TS, Francisco GE, et al. Abrupt withdrawal from intrathecal baclofen: Recognition and management of a potentially life-threatening syndrome. Arch Phys Med Rehabil 2002;83(6):735–41.
31. Flett PJ. Rehabilitation of spasticity and related problems in childhood cerebral palsy. J Paediatr Child Health 2003;39:6–14.
32. Lee M, Alexander MA, Miller F, et al. Postoperative heterotopic ossification in the child with cerebral palsy: three case reports. Arch Phys Med Rehabil 1992;73(3): 289–92.
33. Krum SD, Miller F. Heterotopic ossification after hip and spine surgery in children with cerebral palsy. J Pediatr Orthop 1993;13:739–43.
34. Ma FYP, Selber P, Nattrass GR, et al. Lengthening and transfer of hamstrings for a flexion deformity of the knee in children with bilateral cerebral palsy. Technique and preliminary results. J Bone Joint Surg Br 2006;88:248–54.
35. Chin TYP, Duncan JA, Johnstone BR, et al. Management of the upper limb in cerebral palsy. J Pediatr Orthop B 2005;14:389–404.
36. Presedo A, Oh CW, Dabney KW, et al. Soft-tissue releases to treat spastic hip subluxation in children with cerebral palsy. J Bone Joint Surg Am 2005;87: 832–41.

Index

Note: Page numbers of article titles are in **boldface** type.

A

Abatacept, 239
Acetaminophen, 194
Acupuncture, 205
Adalimumab, 187, 226, 239, 247
Allopurinol, for gout, 188
American College of Rheumatology, juvenile rheumatoid arthritis classification of, 220
Anakinra, 239
Ankle arthrodesis
    complications of, 320–321
    versus total ankle arthroplasty, 300–304
Ankle foot orthosis, 198–200, 229
Ankle joint
    arthrodesis of, 280–287
    arthrodiastasis of, collagen-glycosaminoglycan monolayer with, **327–333**
    arthroplasty of. *See* Total ankle arthroplasty.
    synovectomy of, 279–280
Ankylosing spondylitis, clinical manifestations of, 185
Antibiotics, perioperative, 315
Anticoagulants, for deep vein thrombophlebitis prevention, 239, 307
Antinuclear antibodies, 224
Arthrodesis
    ankle joint, 280–287, 320–321
    first metatarsophalangeal joint, 319
    for metatarsophalangeal joint correction, 255–256
    for midfoot and hindfoot reconstruction, 265–270
    for pediatric patients, 228–229
    for toe pathology, 250
    subtalar joint, collagen-glycosaminoglycan monolayer with, **327–333**
Arthrodiastasis, ankle, collagen-glycosaminoglycan monolayer with, **327–333**
Arthroplasty, 229
    for toe pathology, 250
    silicone implant, in forefoot, 319
    total ankle, 287–288, **295–311,** 321–322
Arthroscopic procedures
    ankle arthrodesis, 285–286
    synovectomy, 279–280
Arthrotomy, mini-, for arthrodesis, 286
Aspirin, 237
Atlantal-axial subluxation, 236–237
Atlizumab, 239
Azathioprine, 239, 247

Clin Podiatr Med Surg 27 (2010) 345–353
doi:10.1016/S0891-8422(10)00019-4

podiatric.theclinics.com

0891-8422/10/$ – see front matter © 2010 Elsevier Inc. All rights reserved.

B

B cells, in rheumatoid arthritis pathophysiology, 277
Balneotherapy, 204–205
Bisphosphonates, 187
Bone remodeling, 276
Bursitis, in midfoot and hindfoot arthritis, 263

C

Calcaneal fractures, subtalar joint arthrodesis for, **327–333**
Calcaneocuboid arthrodesis, 266
Capsulotomy, for digital pathology, 251
Cardiovascular disease, in preoperative evaluation, 190–191
Celecoxib, 186, 194–195, 237
Cerebral palsy, myofascial lengthening for, **335–343**
Cervical spine, rheumatoid arthritis of, 236–237, 246
Chemokine stromal cell-derived factor 1, in rheumatoid arthritis pathophysiology, 279
Chinese medicine, 205
Claw toe, correction of, 249–251
Clayton procedure, for toe pathology, 250
Colchicine, for gout, 188
Cold therapy, 201–202
Collagen-glycosaminoglycan monolayer, for subtalar joint arthrodesis, **327–333**
Complementary and alternative medicine, 204–205
Complications, of surgical treatment, 240–241, **313–325**
    ankle arthrodesis, 320–321
    forefoot, 316–319
    hindfoot, 320
    intraoperative, 315–316
    medication management and, 315
    midfoot and hindfoot reconstruction, 263
    postoperative care and, 316
    preoperative evaluation for, 314–315
    tibiotalocalcaneal arthrodesis, 320–321
    total ankle arthroplasty, 307–308, 321–322
Computed tomography, 214–216
    for midfoot and hindfoot pathology, 263–264
    for pediatric patients, 224
Contrast baths, 201–202
Corticosteroids, 187, 189, 196, 226–227
C-reactive protein, 224
Cyclophosphamide, 239, 247
Cytokines, in rheumatoid arthritis pathophysiology, 276–277

D

Deep vein thrombophlebitis, prevention of, 239, 307
Delayed union, 240
Diclofenac, 194–195
Diet therapy, 204

Digital pathology
    correction of, 249–250
    postoperative, 317–319
Disease-modifying antirheumatic drugs, 187, 195–196, 226, 247

E

Electrophysical modalities, 200–202
Electrotherapy, 202–203
Etanercept, 187, 226, 239, 247
Exercise, 203–204, 229

F

Fasciitis, in midfoot and hindfoot arthritis, 263
Feboxustat, for gout, 188
Fenofibrate, for gout, 188
Fibromyalgia, 185
Fish oil, 204
Footwear modifications, 197–200
Forefoot reconstruction, **243–259**
    combination procedures in, 254–256
    complications of, 316–319
    diagnostic studies for, 244
    digital pathology correction in, 249–252
    imaging for, 244–245
    joint-sparing, 251–254
    medical management with, 245–247
    metatarsophalangeal joint correction in, 252–256
    purpose of, 243–244
    soft tissue removal in, 248–249
Fractures
    calcaneal, subtalar joint arthrodesis for, **327–333**
    malleolar, after total ankle arthroplasty, 307
Fusion. *See* Arthrodesis.

G

Gait analysis, 277–279
Gamma-linolenic acid, 204
Glucocorticoids, 187, 189, 196, 226–227
Gout
    clinical manifestations of, 184–186
    treatment of, 188

H

Hammertoe
    correction of, 249–251
    in midfoot and hindfoot arthritis, 262–263
Healing, postoperative, 314
Heat therapy, 201–202
Herbal therapy, 204

Hibbs procedure
    for forefoot correction, 255–256
    modified, for metatarsophalangeal joint correction, 252–253
Hindfoot reconstruction, **261–273**
    arthrodesis options for, 265–270
    clinical presentation and, 262–263
    complications of, 320
    imaging for, 263–264
    pathophysiologic considerations in, 261–262
    preoperative assessment for, 265
    versus conservative treatment, 264–265
Hoffman procedure, modified, for metatarsophalangeal joint correction, 252–253
Homeopathy, 205
Hydrocortisone, 196, 226–227, 238, 247
Hydrotherapy, 204–205
Hydroxychloroquine, 195, 239

I

Ibuprofen, 186, 195, 237
Imaging, **209–218**. *See also specific modalities.*
    computed tomography, 214–216
    magnetic resonance imaging, 211–213
    of forefoot pathology, 244–245
    of midfoot and hindfoot pathology, 263–264
    radiography, 210–211
    ultrasonography, 213–214
Indomethacin, for gout, 188
Infections, postoperative, 307
Infliximab, 187, 239, 247
Interleukins, in rheumatoid arthritis pathophysiology, 262, 276–277

J

Joint protection, 196–200
Joint replacement, 229. *See also* Total ankle arthroplasty.
Juvenile rheumatoid arthritis, **219–233**
    assessment of, 222–225
    classification of, 220
    clinical manifestations of
        pauciarticular, 220–221
        polyarticular, 221
        systemic, 221–222
    definition of, 219
    pauciarticular, 220–221
    polyarticular, 221
    prevalence of, 220
    prognosis for, 222
    significance of, 220
    subsets of, 220–222
    systemic, 221–222
    treatment of, 226–229

K

Ketorolac, for gout, 188

L

Lapidus procedure, for forefoot correction, 254–256
Laser therapy, low-level, 202
Leflunomide, 187, 239, 247
Leg length discrepancy, 221
Ligamentous laxity syndrome, 185
Losartan, for gout, 188

M

Macrophage activation syndrome, 224
Magnetic resonance imaging, 211–213
    for forefoot pathology, 245
    for midfoot and hindfoot pathology, 263
    for pediatric patients, 224
Malalignment, after total ankle arthroplasty, 307
Malleolar fractures, after total ankle arthroplasty, 307
Mallet toe, correction of, 249–250
Matrix metalloproteases, in rheumatoid arthritis pathophysiology, 279
Meloxicam, 186–187, 194–195
Metatarsal osteotomy, for forefoot correction, 254
Metatarsocuneiform arthrodesis, 266
Metatarsophalangeal joint
    arthrodesis of, 319
    correction of, 252–256
Methotrexate, 195, 226, 238, 247, 315
Methylprednisolone, 196, 238
Midfoot reconstruction, **261–273**
    arthrodesis options for, 265–270
    clinical presentation and, 262–263
    complications of, 320
    imaging for, 263–264
    pathophysiologic considerations in, 261–262
    preoperative assessment for, 265
    versus conservative treatment, 264–265
Mini-arthrotomy, for arthrodesis, 286
Myofascial lengthening, percutaneous, for cerebral palsy, **335–343**

N

Nabumetone, 237
Naproxen, 237
Naviculocuneiform arthrodesis, 266–267
Neuritis, in midfoot and hindfoot arthritis, 263
Neurologic complications, 240
Neuroma, 240

Neuropathic pain, 185
Neuropathy, 240
Nodules, rheumatoid
    differential diagnosis of, 184–185
    in midfoot and hindfoot arthritis, 263
    protective measures for, 197
    removal of, 248–249
Nonsteroidal antiinflammatory drugs, 186–187, 194–195, 226, 237, 247
Nonunion, 240
Nutritional therapy, 204

O

Obstructive sleep apnea, 189
Occupational therapy, 203–204
Orthoses, 197–200, 229
Osteoarthritis, erosive, 185
Osteoblasts, dysfunction of, 277
Osteoclasts, dysfunction of, 276
Osteopenia, 187
Osteotomy, metatarsal, for forefoot correction, 254
Outcome Measures in Rheumatoid Arthritis Clinical Trials, 212–213
Oxaprozin, 237

P

Panmetatarsal head resection, 318–319
Paraffin wax baths, 201
Passive hydrotherapy, 204–205
Pauciarticular juvenile rheumatoid arthritis, 220–221
Pediatric patients
    arthritis in. See Juvenile rheumatoid arthritis.
    cerebral palsy in, selective percutaneous myofascial lengthening for, **335–343**
Penicillamine, 238
Percutaneous procedures
    ankle arthrodesis, 286–287
    myofascial lengthening, for cerebral palsy, **335–343**
Pes planus, in midfoot and hindfoot arthritis, 263
Physical therapy, 203–204, 229
Pin fixation, for metatarsophalangeal joint correction, 252–253
Piroxicam, 237
Plantar fasciitis, 198
Polyarticular juvenile rheumatoid arthritis, 221
Posterior tibial tendon dysfunction, 199–200
Postoperative care, 306–307, 314, 316
Prednisone, 247
    for gout, 188
    for rheumatoid arthritis, 187, 196
Preoperative management, 188–191
    cardiovascular disease evaluation, 190–191
    for complication prevention, 314–315
    of midfoot and hindfoot reconstruction, 265

Probenecid, for gout, 188
Proton pump inhibitors, 186–187

R

Radiography, 210–211
　for forefoot pathology, 244–245
　for midfoot and hindfoot pathology, 263–264
　for pediatric patients, 224
Rau scoring system, 210
Raynaud phenomena, 240
Receptor activator of nuclear factor-κB ligand (RANKL), 276–277
Rheumatoid arthritis
　classification of, 209–210
　clinical manifestations of, 183–186
　　in forefoot, 244
　　in midfoot and hindfoot, 262–263
　　in pediatric patients, 219–225
　conservative treatment of, **193–207**
　　complementary and alternative, 204–205
　　electrotherapy, 202–203
　　exercise, 203–204, 229
　　in midfoot and hindfoot, 264–265
　　joint protective, 196–200
　　pharmacologic, 186–188, 194–196, 226–227, 237–239
　　physical therapy, 203–204, 229
　diagnosis of, 244
　differential diagnosis of, 183–186
　evaluation of, 222–225, **235–241**
　gait analysis in, 277–279
　grading of, 209–210
　imaging for. See Imaging; *specific modalities.*
　juvenile, **219–233**
　osteoimmunology of, 276–277
　pathophysiology of, 261–262, 276–277
　prevalence of, 193–194, 220, 264
　prognosis for, 222
　staging of, 209–210
　surgical treatment of
　　cervical spine disease and, 236–237, 246
　　complications of. See Complications.
　　deep vein thrombophlebitis prevention in, 239, 307
　　efficacy versus effectiveness of, **275–293**
　　forefoot, **243–259,** 316–319
　　in pediatric patients, 227–229
　　laboratory studies for, 239
　　medication review for, 237–239, 315
　　midfoot and hindfoot, **261–273,** 320
　　perioperative management in, **235–241**
　　preoperative considerations for, 188–191, 265, 314–315
　　total ankle arthroplasty, **295–311,** 321–322
　　types of, 189–190

Rheumatoid Arthritis Magnetic Resonance Imaging System, 211–212
Rheumatoid factor, 224
Rofecoxib, 194

S

Scandinavian Total Ankle Replacement implant, 287–288
Selective percutaneous myofascial lengthening, for cerebral palsy, **335–343**
Shoe modifications, 197–200
Silicone implant arthroplasty, in forefoot, 319
Soft tissue release, for pediatric patients, 227
Spa therapy, 204–205
Spasticity, in cerebral palsy, myofascial lengthening for, **335–343**
Steinmann pins, for metatarsophalangeal joint correction, 252
Steroids, 187, 189, 196, 226–227
Subastragaloid arthrodesis, 269
Subtalar joint arthrodesis, collagen-glycosaminoglycan monolayer with, **327–333**
Sulfasalazine, 195, 239, 247
Sulindac, 237
Synovectomy
    ankle joint, 279–280
    for pediatric patients, 227
Synovial fluid examination, 223–224
Synovitis
    clinical manifestations of, 184–185
    imaging of, 212–213
    in midfoot and hindfoot arthritis, 263
Systemic juvenile rheumatoid arthritis, 221–222
Systemic lupus erythematosus, 184

T

T cells, in rheumatoid arthritis pathophysiology, 276–277
Tai chi, 205
Talar dome resurfacing, collagen-glycosaminoglycan monolayer with, **327–333**
Talonavicular arthrodesis, 265–269
Tarsometatarsal arthrodesis, 265–266
Tendon pathology, 240–241
Tenosynovitis, 198–199
Tenotomy, for digital pathology, 251
Thermotherapy, 201
Thrombophlebitis, deep vein, prevention of, 239, 307
Tibiotalocalcaneal arthrodesis, 282–283, 320–321
Tocilizumab, 195
Toe pathology
    correction of, 249–250
    postoperative, 317–319
Total ankle arthroplasty, **295–311**
    background of, 296
    complications of, 307–308, 321–322
    patient selection for, 296–300

postoperative course of, 306–307
technique for, 304–306
versus ankle arthrodesis, 287–288, 300–304
Total joint replacement, 229
Tramadol, 194
Transcutaneous electrical nerve stimulation, 202
Trauma
calcaneal, subtalar joint arthrodesis for, **327–333**
clinical manifestations of, 184
Triamcinolone, 196, 227
Triple arthrodesis, 269–270, 320

U

Ultrasound
diagnostic, 213–214
therapeutic, 201
Union, delayed, 240
Uveitis, 220–221

V

Valdecoxib, 194–195
Vascular complications, 240, 263

W

Weil metatarsal osteotomy, for forefoot correction, 254
Wire fixation, for digital pathology, 251, 254
Wound healing, postoperative, 314